Carol T. Tully
Editor

Lesbian Social Services:
Research Issues

Pre-publication
REVIEWS,
COMMENTARIES,
EVALUATIONS . . .

"**I**n light of the limited body of research which exists on lesbians, this pioneering compilation of articles provides much needed concrete assistance to future researchers. Numerous issues essential to conducting valid and reliable research on a minority such as lesbians are covered in a manner which is both innovative and practical. For example, topics covered include conducting research on older lesbians and ethical dilemmas in conducting research in lesbian communities. The extensive bibliographies will be especially helpful to both practitioners and researchers.

Two timely and important topics discussed, partner abuse in lesbian relationships and fusion and conflict resolution in lesbian relationships, warrant much further research, and the articles in this book will certainly provide a theoretical foundation for such research.

Joyce C. Albro, M.S.W., J.D.

"**H**uman service professionals increasingly recognize the need to increase the knowledge base related to lesbians and gay men. *Lesbian Social Services: Research Issues* is a valuable source book for all social scientists interested in developing their knowledge or doing research in the lesbian community. This volume provides a scholarly, state of the art, analysis of both the methodological and ethical issues that so profoundly shape research for and about lesbians. Through this work, Tully, and the other contributors to the volume, set the standard for future research on and about lesbians. Without question, this important book must be included in the library of every serious scholar of lesbian life, and in the bibliography of social work, counseling, women's studies, and gay studies graduate research courses!

Hilda Hidalgo PhD, ACSW

Professor Emerita Rutgers University

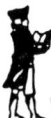

The Haworth Press, Inc.

Lesbian Social Services: Research Issues

Lesbian Social Services: Research Issues

Carol T. Tully, PhD
Editor

Lesbian Social Services: Research Issues, edited by Carol T. Tully, was simultaneously issued by The Haworth Press, Inc., under the same title, as a special issue of *Journal of Gay & Lesbian Social Services*, Volume 3, Number 1 1995, James J. Kelly, Editor.

Harrington Park Press
An Imprint of
The Haworth Press, Inc.
New York · London

1-56023-071-1

Published by

Harrington Park Press, 10 Alice Street, Binghamton, NY 13904-1580 USA

Harrington Park Press is an imprint of The Haworth Press, Inc., 10 Alice Street, Binghamton, NY 13904-1580 USA.

Lesbian Social Services: Research Issues has also been published as *Journal of Gay & Lesbian Social Services,* Volume 3, Number 1 1995.

The development, preparation, and publication of this work has been undertaken with great care. However, the publisher, employees, editors, and agents of The Haworth Press and all imprints of The Haworth Press, Inc., including The Haworth Medical Press and Pharmaceutical Products Press, are not responsible for any errors contained herein or for consequences that may ensue from use of materials or information contained in this work. Opinions expressed by the author(s) are not necessarily those of The Haworth Press, Inc.

Library of Congress Cataloging-in-Publication Data

Lesbian social services: research issues/Carol T. Tully, editor.
     p. cm.
    Includes bibliographical references and index.
    ISBN 1-56024-750-9 (alk. paper). – ISBN 1-56023-071-1 (alk. paper)
     1. Social work with lesbians--Research--United States. 2. Lesbians--Services for--Research--United States. 3. Social service--Research--United States. 4. Gay and lesbian studies--United States. I. Tully, Carol Thorpe, 1946-.
HV1449.L49 1995   95-32130
362.83'9–dc20   CIP

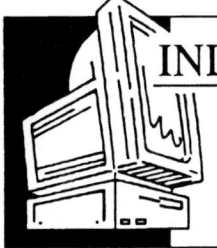# INDEXING & ABSTRACTING

Contributions to this publication are selectively indexed or abstracted in print, electronic, online, or CD-ROM version(s) of the reference tools and information services listed below. This list is current as of the copyright date of this publication. See the end of this section for additional notes.

- *AIDS Newsletter c/o CAB International/CAB ACCESS ...* *available in print, diskettes updated weekly, and on INTERNET. Providing full bibliographic listings, author affiliation, augmented keyword searching,* CAB International, Wallingford Oxon OX10 8DE, United Kingdom

- *Cambridge Scientific Abstracts, Risk Abstracts,* Cambridge Information Group, 7200 Wisconsin Avenue #601, Bethesda, MD 20814

- *caredata CD: the social and community care database,* National Institute for Social Work, 5 Tavistock Place, London WC1H 9SS, England

- *Digest of Neurology and Psychiatry,* The Institute of Living, 400 Washington Street, Hartford, CT 06106

- *ERIC Clearinghouse on Urban Education (ERIC/CUE),* Teachers College, Columbia University, Box 40, New York, NY 10027

- *Family Life Educator "Abstracts Section,"* ETR Associates, P.O. Box 1830, Santa Cruz, CA 95061-1830

- *Homodok,* ILGA Archive, O, Z. Achterburgwal 185, NL-1012, DK Amsterdam, The Netherlands

- *Index to Periodical Articles Related to Law,* University of Texas, 727 East 26th Street, Austin, TX 78705

(continued)

INTERNET ACCESS (& additional networks) Bulletin Board for Libraries ("BUBL"), coverage of information resources on INTERNET, JANET, and other networks.
- JANET X.29: UK.AC.BATH.BUBL or 00006012101300
- TELNET: BUBL.BATH.AC.UK or 138.38.32.45 login 'bubl'
- Gopher: BUBL.BATH.AC.UK (138.32.32.45). Port 70/70
- World Wide Web: http://www.bubl.bath.ac.uk/BUBL/home.html
- NISSWAIS telnetniss.ac.uk (for the NISS gateway)

The Andersonian Library, Curran Building, 101 St. James Road, Glasgow G4 ONS, Scotland

- *Inventory of Marriage and Family Literature (online and hard copy),* National Council on Family Relations, 3989 Central Avenue NE, Suite 550, Minneapolis, MN 55421

- *Mental Health Abstracts (online through DIALOG),* IFI/Plenum Data Company, 3202 Kirkwood Highway, Wilmington, DE 19808

- *Referativnyi Zhurnal (Abstracts Journal of the Institute of Scientific Information of the Republic of Russia),* The Institute of Scientific Information, Baltijskaja ul., 14, Moscow A-219, Republic of Russia

- *Social Work Abstracts,* National Association of Social Workers, 750 First Street NW, 8th Floor, Washington, DC 20002

- *Sociological Abstracts (SA),* Sociological Abstracts, Inc., P.O. Box 22206, San Diego, CA 92192-0206

- *Studies on Women Abstracts,* Carfax Publishing Company, P.O. Box 25, Abingdon, Oxfordshire OX14 3UE, United Kingdom

- *Violence and Abuse Abstracts: A Review of Current Literature on Interpersonal Violence (VAA),* Sage Publications, Inc., 2455 Teller Road, Newbury Park, CA 91320

(continued)

SPECIAL BIBLIOGRAPHIC NOTES

related to special journal issues (separates)
and indexing/abstracting

- [ ] indexing/abstracting services in this list will also cover material in any "separate" that is co-published simultaneously with Haworth's special thematic journal issue or DocuSerial. Indexing/abstracting usually covers material at the article/chapter level.

- [ ] monographic co-editions are intended for either non-subscribers or libraries which intend to purchase a second copy for their circulating collections.

- [ ] monographic co-editions are reported to all jobbers/wholesalers/approval plans. The source journal is listed as the "series" to assist the prevention of duplicate purchasing in the same manner utilized for books-in-series.

- [ ] to facilitate user/access services all indexing/abstracting services are encouraged to utilize the co-indexing entry note indicated at the bottom of the first page of each article/chapter/contribution.

- [ ] this is intended to assist a library user of any reference tool (whether print, electronic, online, or CD-ROM) to locate the monographic version if the library has purchased this version but not a subscription to the source journal.

- [ ] individual articles/chapters in any Haworth publication are also available through the Haworth Document Delivery Services (HDDS).

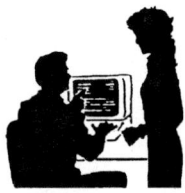

CONTENTS

ABOUT THE EDITOR

CAROL T. TULLY, PhD, MSW, is Associate Professor and Director of Field Instruction in the School of Social Work at Tulane University. She has published articles, book chapters, and educational guides and has been involved in organizing or presenting at a number of professional and learned societies. Dr. Tully serves on the editorial boards of the *Journal of Gay & Lesbian Psychotherapy,* the *Journal of Gay & Lesbian Social Services,* the *Journal of Gay and Lesbian Health,* and the *Journal of Social Work Education.*

Foreword

The lesbian and gay experience has been explored in an ever-growing body of research studies and fiction since the landmark Stonewall riots energized a national gay rights movement more than two decades ago. For many people, "coming out of the closet" has become a critical step in development of mature self-identity. Books and studies have been published on sexual orientation, institutionalized and internalized homophobia, and developmental phases of same-sex relationships. Those works, along with many self-help manuals and fiction, have contributed to the development of lesbian and gay community identity, and to the self-concept of lesbian women and gay men.

And yet, and yet. In this area of research and writing, as in so many others, there is a curious and abiding discrepancy. Whether one reviews academic research, or popular gay oriented magazines, or fiction, lesbians are underrepresented, overlooked, in the shadows, or invisible and left out.

Why is this? The simplest–and probably most accurate–reason is that lesbians are subject to double discrimination. Both homophobia and sexism can be implicated. Scholarly exploration of lesbian issues has not been encouraged in academe. Indeed, some courageous writers have been denigrated by peers for devoting so much energy to a subject deemed to be frivolous, and certainly detrimental to progress along the increasingly difficult road to tenure.

Carol Tully and her colleagues have taken a major step toward increasing our knowledge about the experiences, relationships and

[Haworth co-indexing entry note]: "Foreword." Lloyd, Gary A. Co-published simultaneously in *Journal of Gay & Lesbian Social Services* (The Haworth Press, Inc.) Vol. 3, No. 1, 1995, pp. xiii-xiv; and: *Lesbian Social Services: Research Issues* (ed: Carol T. Tully) The Haworth Press, Inc., 1995, pp. xi-xii; and: *Lesbian Social Services: Research Issues* (ed: Carol T. Tully) Harrington Park Press, an imprint of The Haworth Press, Inc., 1995, pp. xi-xii. Multiple copies of this article/chapter may be purchased from The Haworth Document Delivery Center [1-800-3-HAWORTH; 9:00 a.m. - 5:00 p.m. (EST)].

xi

concerns of lesbians. By focusing on research issues, the editor and authors heighten awareness about lesbianism at the same time they demonstrate research strategies and methodological approaches to the study of a large and virtually ignored group of women in the United States.

The work presented here ranges widely from affirmative psychotherapy to methodological issues, on to relationship concerns and ethical dilemmas in conducting research in lesbian communities. A common theme is the difficulty in locating samples from a population which is often afraid to be made visible because of stereotyping, stigma and discrimination.

These six papers are extremely valuable and timely contributions to the emerging field of lesbian studies. One can only hope that the rich and varied work of Carol Tully and her associates will inspire others to engage in research and writing about lesbianism. Otherwise, lesbians will continue to be rendered invisible by the double stigma, and a potentially exciting and vital opportunity for research on developmental issues, sexuality, sexual orientation, and social policy will be lost.

Gary A. Lloyd, PhD, ACSW
School of Social Work
Tulane University

Preface

This volume emerged from my discussions at learned society meetings and academic settings with colleagues and students about the state of the art of lesbian research. We all agreed that research about lesbians was an often overlooked, but fertile area for exploration. We further concluded that, to date, no one had systematically sought to specifically identify research issues related to gathering data on an invisible minority whose only common characteristic was sexual orientation. We also recognized that research in the area of lesbianism was still considered fairly unpopular, but were encouraged by the recent trend in the social sciences to accept lesbian and gay studies as a legitimate area of scholarship. So, it was with this background I came to select the research oriented theme of this volume.

Conceptualized around major topics of a research study, this volume provides an examination of the current state of the art, methodological issues, and ethical dilemmas associated with conducting research using lesbians. Divided into six papers, ten scholars in the area of lesbian studies have provided pragmatic ideas and support for others who wish to conduct research using lesbian samples. The first paper provides a literature review of research about lesbians and lesbianism from 1950-1990. It identifies five major phases of lesbian research: etiology, psychological functioning, social functioning, life span development, and clinical intervention. Papers two, three, and four specifically explore methodological issues germane to this population. Building on the emerging para-

[Haworth co-indexing entry note]: "Preface." Tully, Carol T. Co-published simultaneously in *Journal of Gay & Lesbian Social Services* (The Haworth Press, Inc.) Vol. 3, No. 1, 1995, pp. xv-xvi; and: *Lesbian Social Services: Research Issues* (ed: Carol T. Tully) The Haworth Press, Inc., 1995, pp. xiii-xiv; and: *Lesbian Social Services: Research Issues* (ed: Carol T. Tully) Harrington Park Press, an imprint of The Haworth Press, Inc., 1995, pp. xiii-xiv. Multiple copies of this article/chapter may be purchased from The Haworth Document Delivery Center [1-800-3-HAWORTH; 9:00 a.m. - 5:00 p.m. (EST)].

xiii

digm shift from oppressive to affirmative psychotherapy for the lesbian woman and the gay man, the second paper presents an excellent analysis of the utility of single-system research designs for evaluating affirmative psychotherapy with lesbians and gay men. Paper three presents a well-articulated case for use of the feminist participatory research model in studying partner abuse in lesbian relationships. The benefits of the feminist model are examined in the context of allowing the members of an invisible and oppressed minority to shape the research about themselves and by allowing researchers to become learners during the research process. In the fourth paper, methodological issues associated with conducting research with older lesbians and research in minority communities are clearly addressed. Paper five skillfully addresses three areas in which professional ethical dilemmas can arise when conducting research with lesbians: confidentiality, anonymity, and professional boundaries. Future researchers may find the proposed solutions to these dilemmas helpful. Finally, the last paper presents a study that used a lesbian sample to explore issues of social distancing and conflict resolution in lesbian relationships. Each of the papers has excellent reference lists that should help the novice and the experienced scholar continue the development of research that provides valid and reliable data on and about lesbians. The authors and the women they have studied make this volume a reality and they, along with my editor, my partner, and future social scientists are the reason this work exists.

Carol T. Tully, PhD
New Orleans

In Sickness and in Health:
Forty Years of Research on Lesbians

Carol T. Tully

SUMMARY. Research about lesbians and lesbianism has only been conducted in a systematic fashion since the 1950s. This article identifies the five major phases of lesbian research: (1) etiology, (2) psychological functioning, (3) social functioning, (4) life span development, and (5) clinical intervention. In addition, the author traces the historical development of the literature for the past four decades.

It is unknown how many homosexuals currently exist in the United States, much less how many of that number are women. Estimates on the size of the American homosexual community vary from 26 million, or about 10% of the total population (Kinsey, Pomeroy, & Martin, 1948; Kinsey, Pomeroy, Martin, & Gebhard, 1953), to 8 million or about 3% of the population (National Opinion Research Center, 1989-1992; Rogers, 1993). Given these figures, a conservative estimate is that between 4 million and 13.5 million lesbians currently live in the United States. Although lesbians do compose a significant minority population, research on any aspect of lesbianism has only been attempted in this country in a systematic fashion since the mid-1950s and consists of five major research

Carol T. Tully, PhD, is Associate Professor at Tulane School of Social Work, Tulane University, New Orleans, LA 70118-5672.

[Haworth co-indexing entry note]: "In Sickness and in Health: Forty Years of Research on Lesbians." Tully, Carol T. Co-published simultaneously in *Journal of Gay & Lesbian Social Services* (The Haworth Press, Inc.) Vol. 3, No. 1, 1995, pp. 1-18; and: *Lesbian Social Services: Research Issues* (ed: Carol T. Tully) The Haworth Press, Inc., 1995, pp. 1-18; and: *Lesbian Social Services: Research Issues* (ed: Carol T. Tully) Harrington Park Press, an imprint of The Haworth Press, Inc., 1995, pp. 1-18. Multiple copies of this article/chapter may be purchased from The Haworth Document Delivery Center [1-800-3-HAWORTH; 9:00 a.m. - 5:00 p.m. (EST)].

phases that span the past four decades. Research across this time span includes data on the etiology of lesbianism, the psychological functioning of lesbian women, the social functioning of lesbians, life span development of lesbians, and professional intervention with lesbians and their families. In the literature review presented in this article, the author analyzes each research trend and provides a historical examination of research on lesbians since its inception.

ETIOLOGY

The first phase of lesbian research, begun in the 1950s and conducted primarily by men, dealt almost exclusively with the question of lesbian etiology. Such research continued sparsely through the 1960s and 1970s and tended to vanish during the 1980s, only to reappear in the 1990s. Of the five broad topic areas listed in Epstein and Zak's (1992) extensive annotated bibliography that examined the literature from 1986 to 1991, etiology was not included. As a group, those studies that dealt with the causation of lesbianism tended to fall into two broad categories: those that dealt with clinical samples and those that did not. Both clinical and nonclinical studies fell into four major areas: (1) socialization and role identification during childhood, (2) parental relationships, (3) family history, and (4) genetics.

Regarding the socialization and role identification process, some researchers have agreed that lesbians may be socialized differently than heterosexual women (Poole, 1970; Thompson, 1971). Furthermore, some researchers believe that lesbians either lack the role learning experiences that heterosexual women had during childhood (Poole, 1970) or that the parents of lesbians interfered with their daughters' role learning experiences (Kay et al., 1967).

In studies that explored parental relationships, data indicated that lesbians tended to have less satisfying relationships with both parents than did heterosexual women (Kay et al., 1967; Kenyon, 1969; Poole, 1970; Siegelman, 1974; Swanson, Loomis, Lukesh, Cornin, & Smith, 1972; Thompson, McCandless, & Strickland, 1971); however, some of the data were contradictory. For example, regarding family history, data showed disagreement about whether there was any significant relationship between birth order and lesbianism

(Gundlach & Riess, 1967; Kenyon, 1968). Data also revealed more separation, divorce, and family discord in the families of lesbians (Kenyon, 1968; Poole, 1970; Swanson, Loomis, Lukesh, Cornin, & Smith, 1972) and more homosexuals in the biological families of homosexual women than in similar families of heterosexual women (Kenyon, 1968).

Overall, to date, research on the etiology of lesbianism has proven contradictory and inconclusive. Although studies of the 1970s indicated that lesbianism was an acquired trait as opposed to an innate one, Bell, Weinberg, and Hammersmith (1981) concluded, on the basis of in-depth, face-to-face interviews with 686 gay men and 293 lesbians, that homosexuality may be more innate than earlier research demonstrated. Hence, Bell, Weinberg and Hammersmith (1981) reintroduced the possibility of a biological foundation for homosexuality that was first suggested in the mid-1800s, became a popular belief in the latter part of the 19th century, and gradually declined as a theory when it was replaced by the psychoanalytic theories of the early 1900s. Interestingly, through the work of Bailey, Pillard, Neale, and Agyei (1991), LeVay (1991), and others (see De Cecco & Elia, 1993), who reintroduced the idea of a genetic component to homosexuality, the etiology of lesbianism is again becoming a focal point for emerging research.

PSYCHOLOGICAL FUNCTIONING

The second major phase of research dealing with lesbians sought to explore lesbian personality and psychological functioning. Research compiled by both women and men between the 1960s and 1980s focused on comparisons between non-clinical samples of lesbian and heterosexual women and sought to determine if lesbianism constituted psychopathology. Such research on the psychological functioning of lesbians supported the idea that lesbian and non-lesbian women had different personality characteristics (Freedman, 1967; Hassell & Smith, 1975; Hopkins, 1969; Ohlson & Wilson, 1974; Thompson, McCandless, & Strickland, 1971; Wilson & Greene, 1971). However, these data were contradictory as to whether identified differences constituted lesbian pathology (Kenyon, 1968). Most of these early studies found lesbian samples or matched lesbian-heterosexual women samples to be psychologically healthy and psychodynamically similar (Armon, 1960; Freedman, 1967; Hopkins, 1969; Miranda & Storms, 1989; Ohlson & Wilson, 1974; Siegelman, 1972; Wilson & Greene, 1971). In general, personality traits that seem to distinguish the lesbian from her nonlesbian counterpart are the lesbian's higher capacity for self-confidence, self-sufficiency, dominance, assertiveness, aggressiveness, and independence (Thompson, McCandless, & Strickland, 1971; Wilson & Greene, 1971).

Following the traditional medical model, such early studies of lesbian psychological functioning assumed that gross differences would exist between heterosexual and homosexual women and that such differences would constitute psychological pathology in the lesbian; these assumptions were unsupported by the data. This phase of viewing the lesbian as an abnormal pathological entity has yielded to the more current trend of conducting psychological research on lesbians that is based on an exploration of the lesbian's functioning from a normal, psychologically healthy perspective.

Once homosexuality was removed from the list of diagnostic mental disorders by the American Psychiatric Association (APA), lesbian psychological research that evolved in the 1970s (and continues to date) tended to explore the development of the lesbian personality from a more positive perspective. Written primarily by women, these more current studies have examined models of identity development (Cass, 1979; Chan, 1989; Chapman & Brannock, 1987; Kahn, 1991; Klein, Sepekoff, & Wolf, 1985; Lewis, 1984; Reiter, 1989; Sophie, 1985/1986). In addition, for the first time, researchers explored lesbianism from a multicultural perspective (Chan, 1989; Loiacano, 1989; Lukes & Land, 1990). Researchers also seemed to agree that lesbians develop and integrate their lesbian identities in identifiable developmental stages (Cass, 1979; Chapman & Brannock, 1987; Kahn, 1991; Lewis, 1984; Sophie, 1985/1986), and that lesbianism includes far more than merely a sexual act (Cass, 1979; Klein, Sepekoff, & Wolf, 1985; Lewis, 1984; Reiter, 1989). The new psychologically-based research on lesbians also has included data on ethnic minorities that showed that nonwhite lesbians face special psychological challenges including racism, sexism, and homophobia as they develop their lesbian identities (Chan, 1989; Loiacano, 1989; Lukes & Land, 1990).

Overall, the research on the psychological functioning of lesbian women has followed the historical trend of moving from a model that explored pathology and abnormality to one of health and normalcy. Although lesbian behavior is not universally accepted as normal, current researchers, like those studying social functioning, are collecting data from psychologically healthy, socially involved, and active lesbians.

SOCIAL FUNCTIONING

During the 1970s, increasing research on lesbians and their social functioning began to appear. This research, done primarily by lesbians, explored lesbian women as psychologically healthy individuals and began to fill in gaps created by the earlier research. Studies on social functioning constitute the third major phase of lesbian research. Roughly divided into three major areas–(1) lesbian characteristics, (2) social functioning, and (3) sexuality–these studies provided the foundation for the work that followed in the 1980s and 1990s.

Generally descriptive, the studies related to personal characteristics depicted lesbians as young, well-educated, professionals who had been involved with few partners and who were in long-term monogamous relationships (Belote & Joesting, 1976; Cotten, 1975; Gagnon & Simon, 1973; Gundlach, 1967; Saghir & Robins, 1969). Although data suggested that lesbians may have higher incidence of substance abuse than heterosexual women (Swanson, Loomis, Lukesh, Cornin, & Smith, 1972) and conflicts around jealousy (Mendola, 1980), those lesbians sampled during the 1970s overwhelmingly accepted themselves as lesbians and were content with their sexual orientation (Albro & Tully, 1979; Belote & Joesting, 1976; Califia, 1979; Gagnon & Simon, 1973; Saghir & Robins, 1969). Other data indicated that the lesbians of the 1970s did not ordinarily play male/female (butch/femme) roles (Belote & Joesting, 1976; Lewis, 1980; Saghir & Robins, 1969; Tripp, 1976), but that some may have played such roles at some point in their lives (Mendola, 1980; Tanner, 1978; Tripp, 1976).

Those studies that examined social functioning suggested that lesbians interacted well in the heterosexual culture, where they gained economic support through professional employment, and in the homosexual subculture where they found emotional support, friendship groups, and an extended family (Albro & Tully, 1979; Chafetz, Sampson, Beck, & West, 1974; Chafetz, Sampson, Beck, West, & Jones, 1976; Gagnon & Simon, 1973; Lewis, 1980; Mendola, 1980; Ponse, 1978; Tanner, 1978). Data further demonstrated that lesbians did not view the heterosexual culture as being accepting of their lifestyle (Albro & Tully, 1979; Belote & Joesting, 1976; Bullough & Bullough, 1977; Chafetz, Sampson, Beck, & West, 1974; Chafetz, Sampson, Beck, West, & Jones, 1976; Gagnon & Simon, 1973; Ponse, 1978), which may have caused them stress (Albro & Tully, 1979; Bullough & Bullough, 1977; Chafetz, Sampson, Beck, & West, 1974; Chafetz, Sampson, Beck, West, & Jones, 1976; Gagnon & Simon, 1973). Although these studies tended to support the idea that lesbians functioned adequately in both the heterosexual and homosexual worlds (Albro & Tully, 1979; Lewis, 1980; Martin, 1960), the data also showed that many lesbians, at some point in their lives, had sought professional counseling (Albro & Tully, 1979; Chafetz, Sampson, Beck, & West, 1974; Chafetz, Sampson, Beck, West, & Jones, 1976).

Although the lesbian subculture has been characterized by these studies as providing lesbians with a social network, a sense of identification, and ideology, and most lesbians found a social support system within the homosexual subculture, some lesbians isolated themselves from the lesbian subculture (Albro & Tully, 1979; Ettorre, 1980; Lewis, 1980). Also, many lesbians apparently resisted publicly acknowledging their sexual orientation (Belote & Joesting, 1976; Bullough & Bullough, 1977; Chafetz, Sampson, Beck, & West, 1974; Chafetz, Sampson, Beck, West, & Jones, 1976; Ettorre, 1980; Gagnon & Simon, 1973; Lewis, 1980; Martin, 1960; Ponse, 1978), and most lesbians were constrained to "pass" as heterosexuals at various times throughout their lives (Albro & Tully, 1979; Bullough & Bullough, 1977; Chafetz, Sampson, Beck, & West, 1974; Chafetz, Sampson, Beck, West, & Jones, 1976; Ettorre, 1980; Lewis, 1980; Martin, 1960; Ponse, 1978; Weinberg, 1973). Yet, during the 1970s, there was growing evidence of a gradually increasing block of politically active lesbians who were beginning to challenge the structure of the traditional heterosexual culture (Ettorre, 1980; Lewis, 1980).

The data also demonstrated that lesbians tended to have a large repertoire of sexual behaviors, appeared sexually active, and were sexually satisfied (Califia, 1979; Kinsey, Pomeroy, Martin, & Gebhard, 1953; Saghir & Robins, 1969). Moreover, although early studies indicated that lesbians had a strong tendency to be emotionally involved with their sexual partners (Davis, 1929; Gagnon & Simon, 1973), a later study indicated that such emotional involvement may not be needed for a satisfactory sexual liaison (Califia, 1979).

The 1970s provided the foundation for studies related to social functioning that followed in the 1980s and 1990s. The recurring themes of family interaction and parental influence found primarily in the early stage of research on lesbians (Gundlach & Riess, 1967; Kay et al., 1967; Kenyon, 1969; Poole, 1970) were evidenced in fewer subsequent studies (Murphy, 1989; Savin-Williams, 1989b; Strommen, 1989), and new themes related to cultural issues (Cochran & Mays, 1986; Kanuha, 1990; Morales, 1989), disability (Doucette, 1989; Sorella, 1991-1992), and other social issues related to being a lesbian (Berrill, 1990; Dworkin, 1988; Ficarrotto, 1990; Modrcin & Wyers, 1990; Post, 1991; Ritter & O'Neill, 1989; Saunders & Valente, 1987) became a primary research focus.

Studies related to family interaction and parental influences tended to push the boundaries of knowledge, and rather than merely examine only the lesbian within the context of the family, researchers examined the family itself as the unit of analysis. For example, Strommen (1989) studied family members' reactions to the disclosure of homosexuality and identified stages that families go through in accepting the gay or lesbian member. Savin-Williams (1989b) examined parental influences on the self-esteem of 317 gay and lesbian youths, and Murphy (1989) gathered data on parental attitudes of the lesbian's family of origin toward her family of choice.

Studies on lesbians who were also members of a minority group became increasingly evident in the 1980s. Several studies explored social supports, families, and oppression of lesbians of color (Cochran & Mays, 1986; Kanuha, 1990; Morales, 1989) or provided information on lesbians with disabilities (Doucette, 1989; Sorella, 1991-1992). These studies generally depicted the lesbian who is also a member of another minority group, as being oppressed because of her sex, sexuality, and other minority status, placing her at risk of discrimination from the society at large, her subculture, and her family (Cochran & Mays, 1986; Doucette, 1989; Morales, 1989; Sorella, 1991-1992).

In addition to studies related to families or minority status, researchers during the 1980s and early 1990s began to focus on the impact of societal values on lesbians and the communities in which they lived. Homophobia and the violence it can spawn (Berrill, 1990; Ficarrotto, 1990; Hooks, 1988), suicide risk among lesbians and gay men (Saunders & Valente, 1987), body image (Dworkin, 1988), maintaining a sense of identity in a homophobic setting (Post, 1991), and spirituality (Ritter & O'Neill, 1989) became research issues.

In summary, research that explored the social functioning of lesbians had its origins in the 1970s with studies that gathered data on lesbian characteristics, social interactions, and sexuality. These primarily descriptive studies, conducted by lesbians themselves, provided the standard by which the studies of the 1980s and 1990s were developed. Moving from the data of the 1970s that described primarily white, middle-class lesbians, more recent data have examined the social functioning of a culturally diverse spectrum of lesbians.

LIFE SPAN DEVELOPMENT

Research that focused on issues related to the life span development of lesbians began in the 1980s and continues today. Divided roughly into areas that mirror the life span–childhood, adolescence, early adulthood, midlife, and aging–these studies have provided another view of lesbians.

Little research exists on when an individual becomes a homosexual. Recent data have tended to support a genetic basis for sexual orientation (Bailey, Pillard, Neal, & Agyei, 1991; LeVay, 1991), but how and when an individual becomes a lesbian needs much more study. A few studies, though, have been conducted on issues associated with puberty and lesbianism (Hersch, 1991; Hetrick & Martin, 1987; Rofes, 1983; Savin-Williams, 1989a; Schneider,

1989) and have examined developmental issues for adolescents (Hetrick & Martin, 1987; Savin-Williams, 1989a, 1989b; Schneider, 1989), support groups (Robinson, 1991), suicide risk (Rofes, 1983), and therapeutic intervention with lesbian and gay adolescents (Coleman & Remafedi, 1989). Such work has provided the first empirical data on adolescent lesbians and gays. Perhaps because of the sensitive nature of gathering data on children and teenagers, a greater focus has been placed on conducting research using adults as the unit of analysis.

Studies that gathered data on lesbians in early adulthood, midlife, and old age have completed the life span studies of the 1980s and 1990s. Data collected on lesbians in early adulthood have added to the previous work by providing descriptive data on couples (Cherry & Mitulski, 1990), parenting (Gibbs, 1989; Gottman, 1989; Levy, 1992; Lott-Whitehead & Tully, 1993; Turner, Scadden, & Harris, 1990; Wyers, 1987) and career development (Post, 1991). Although fewer in number, studies on midlife lesbians have explored social support systems (Tully, 1989) and career counseling (Hetherington & Orzek, 1989). Furthermore, lesbian gerontological issues have become the focus of recent study (Friend, 1989; Galassi, 1991; Kehoe, 1988; Poor, 1982).

Data on older lesbians became the focus of a few researchers at the start of the 1980s and, perhaps due to the rapidly growing older population and the lack of data before 1980, became an emerging field of study. As with most of the research, those studies for which data were collected using a survey tended to be cross-sectional and descriptive. Also, samples generally were obtained using a snowball sampling technique. Consequently, the results tended to portray older lesbians as well-educated, white, middle-class women who may or may not have ever married and were in good-to-excellent emotional and physical health, even though they may have had chronic medical problems. Furthermore, older lesbians were depicted as being actively involved with life, and maintaining a series of relationships and social activities with those their own age. Although some may have lost a partner, and many lived alone, most have maintained a high degree of satisfaction with life (Friend, 1989; Kehoe, 1988; Poor, 1982; Tully, 1983).

As with other types of research, the studies related to lesbian life span development and the issues associated with aging have tended to confirm previous data in the field of lesbianism: simply, that lesbians, because of their sexual orientation, face unique problems as they age, but seem to develop healthy relationships and coping mechanisms, and maintain social interactions throughout their lives.

PROFESSIONAL INTERVENTION WITH LESBIANS

An area of research that recently has attracted the most attention and that is closely related to the literature on psychological functioning of lesbians is the provision of professional social services to lesbians. Rather than focusing on clinical issues that separate lesbians from their heterosexual counterparts (as did the studies of the 1960s and 1970s), research of the 1980s and 1990s has examined clinical intervention from the standpoint of assessment, specific therapeutic issues, and ethics. The focus of current studies has changed from one of pathology to one of trying to help lesbians live a psychologically healthy life.

Few authors have chosen to examine issues associated with the clinical assessment of lesbians; those who have, though, have explored the issue in terms of what precipitates lesbian clients to seek help (Modrcin & Wyers, 1990), theoretical issues associated with assessment (Stein, 1983), cultural or personal homophobia as a deterrent to appropriate assessment with lesbian clients (Cohen & Stein, 1986; Seigel, 1987; Smith, 1988), and general overviews of the assessment process (Hidalgo, Peterson, & Woodman, 1985; Kus, 1990; Shernoff & Scott, 1988; Woodman, 1992).

Of more interest to researchers seems to be special issues associated with lesbian clients in therapy. No longer characterized by the APA as a pathology, since the late 1970s, lesbianism has been the focus of research on unique therapeutic issues associated with being a member of an oppressed minority group. Additionally, therapists are beginning to examine their role in the therapeutic process with lesbians and gay men.

In addition to an examination of general clinical issues associated with the psychological health of lesbians (Garnets, Hancock, Cochran, Goodchilds, & Peplau, 1991; Woodman, 1988), recent research also has examined clinical issues associated with codependency of lesbian couples (Finnegan & McNally, 1988; Smalley, 1987), family of origin issues (Brown, 1989), and lesbians as victims of crime (Wertheimer, 1990), sexual assault (Orzek, 1988) or lesbian battering (Morrow & Hawxhurst, 1989). Furthermore, data have tended to indicate that perhaps internalized homophobia is associated with substance abuse in lesbians. Researchers who have collected data on issues associated with lesbians and substance abuse (Anderson & Henderson, 1985; Faltz, 1988; Finnegan & McNally, 1988; Glaus, 1989) seem to agree that there may be a disproportionate number of lesbians who have substance abuse problems than is found in the general heterosexual population. In addition to substance abuse, depression (Rothblum, 1990) and neurosis (Cabaj, 1989) in lesbians may, too, have their roots in homophobia. Although most of the clinical research of the 1980s and 1990s has tended to focus on psychopathology, at least one author examined lesbianism as a positive lifestyle model for women (Rothblum, 1988).

Other authors have chosen to examine issues that assure appropriate therapeutic intervention with lesbians. For example, Greene (1986) provided data about white heterosexual therapists working with lesbian and heterosexual African-American women, and Schwartz (1988) examined therapeutic interventions involving a homosexual therapist and a nonhomosexual client. Markowitz (1991) argued that therapists are generally still ill-equipped to deal with lesbian and gay clients, and McDermott, Tyndall and Lichtenberg's (1989) data tended to support the idea that lesbian and gay clients prefer lesbian or gay therapists. Buhrke (1988) addressed issues related to lesbianism in counseling supervision, and the first work in the area of ethics and lesbianism emerged in the late 1980s (Brown, 1988; Sobocinski, 1990).

Recent trends in clinical intervention with lesbians, then, have moved from trying to identify pathology as a result of homosexuality to pathology as a result of institutionalized homophobia and societal stressors placed on the lesbian. In addition, clinical intervention has moved away from curing the lesbian of her homosexuality to helping her cope with presenting problems beyond sexual orientation issues.

CONCLUSIONS

A significant amount of research that provided data about lesbians and lesbianism has been conducted since the 1950s and into the 1990s. The focus of this research shifted from lesbianism as a pathology to lesbianism as an alternative lifestyle. Early studies about lesbianism conducted primarily by men using the psychoanalytic framework, gave way to research conducted by women, who have more frequently used feminist theory as their conceptual framework. Generally, during the past four decades, there has been a continuing sharpening of focus on studies dealing with lesbians: current studies have not examined lesbians as a homogeneous group, but rather, as a heterogeneous group as diverse as the American population. This broader focus certainly allows for a more realistic view of lesbians and will undoubtedly continue into the 21st century. Because data in this field of study are still relatively sparse, it is an excellent area to pursue for those interested in providing empirical evidence to refute the continuing mythology about lesbians and lesbianism.

REFERENCES

Albro, J. C., & Tully, C. T. (1979). A study of lesbian lifestyles in the homosexual micro-culture and the heterosexual macro-culture. *Journal of Homosexuality, 4*(4), 331-344.

Anderson, S. C., & Henderson, D. C. (1985). Working with lesbian alcoholics. *Social Work, 30*(6), 518-525.

Armon, V. (1960). Some personality variables in overt female homosexuality. *Journal of Projective Technique of Personality Assessment, 24*(3), 292-309.

Bailey, J. M., Pillard, R. C., Neale, M. C., & Agyei, Y. (1991). Heritable factors influence sexual orientation in women. *Archives of General Psychiatry, 50*(3), 217-223.

Bell, A. P., Weinberg, M. S., & Hammersmith, S. K. (1981). *Sexual preference.* Bloomington: Indiana University Press.

Belote, D., & Joesting, J. (1976). Demographic and self-report characteristics of lesbians. *Psychological Reports, 39,* 621-622.

Berrill, K. T. (1990). Anti-gay violence and victimization in the United States. *Journal of Interpersonal Violence, 5*(3), 274-294.

Brown, L. S. (1988). Beyond thou shalt not: Thinking about ethics in the lesbian therapy community. *Women & Therapy, 8*(1/2), 13-25.

Brown, L. S. (1989). Lesbian, gay men and their families: Common clinical issues. *Journal of Gay & Lesbian Psychotherapy, 1*(1), 37-53.

Buhrke, R. A. (1988). Lesbian-related issues in counseling supervision. *Women & Therapy, 8*(1/2), 195-206.

Bullough, V. L., & Bullough, B. (1977). Lesbianism in the 1920s and 1930s: A newfound study. *Signs, 2*(4), 895-904.

Cabaj, R. P. (1989). Homosexuality and neurosis: Considerations for psychotherapy. In M. W. Ross (Ed.), *Psychopathology and psychotherapy in homosexuality* (pp. 13-23). Binghamton, NY: The Haworth Press, Inc.

Califia, P. (1979). Lesbian sexuality. *Journal of Homosexuality, 4*(3), 255-266.

Cass, V. C. (1979). Homosexual identity formation: A theoretical model. *Journal of Homosexuality, 4*(3), 219-235.

Chafetz, J. S., Sampson, P., Beck, P., & West, J. (1974). A study of homosexual women. *Social Work, 19*(6), 714-723.

Chafetz, J. S., Sampson, P., Beck, P., West, J., & Jones, B. (1976). *Who's queer: A study of homo and heterosexual women.* Sarasota, FL: Omni Press.

Chan, C. S. (1989). Issues of identity development among Asian-American lesbians and gay men. *Journal of Counseling and Development, 68*(1), 16-20.

Chapman, B. E., & Brannock, J. C. (1987). Proposed model of lesbian identity development: An empirical examination. *Journal of Homosexuality, 14*(3/4), 69-80.

Cherry, K., & Mitulski, J. (1990). Committed couples in the gay community. *Christian Century, 107*(7), 218-220.

Cochran, S. D., & Mays, V. M. (1986, August). *Sources of support in the black lesbian community.* Paper presented at the annual meeting of the American Psychological Association, Washington, DC.

Cohen, C. J., & Stein, T. S. (1986). Reconceptualizing individual psychotherapy with gay men and lesbians. In T. S. Stein & C. J. Cohen (Eds.), *Contemporary perspectives on psychotherapy with lesbians and gay men* (pp. 27-54). New York: Plenum Medical Book.

Coleman, E., & Remafedi, G. (1989). Gay, lesbian, and bisexual adolescents: A critical challenge to counselors. *Journal of Counseling and Development, 68*(1), 36-40.

Cotten, W. L. (1975). Social and sexual relationships of lesbians. *Journal of Sex Research, 11,* 139-148.

Davis, K. B. (1929). *Factors in the sex life of twenty-two hundred women.* New York: Harper.

De Cecco, J. P., & Elia, J. P. (Eds.). (1993). If you seduce a straight person, can you make them gay? Issues in biological essentialism versus social constructionism in gay and lesbian identities [Special issue]. *Journal of Homosexuality, 24*(3).

Doucette, J. (1989). Redefining difference: Disabled lesbians resist. *Resources for Feminist Research, 18*(2), 17-21.

Dworkin, S. H. (1988). Not in man's image: Lesbians and the cultural oppression of body image. *Women & Therapy, 8*(1/2), 27-39.

Epstein, A. L., & Zak, P. D. (1992). *The master of social work core curriculum:*

Inclusion of gay, lesbian and bisexual content–An annotated bibliography. San Francisco: Author.

Ettorre, E. M. (1980). *Lesbians, women and society.* Boston: Routledge & Kegan Paul.

Faltz, B. G. (1988). Substance abuse in the lesbian and gay community: Assessment and intervention. In M. Shernoff & W. A. Scott (Eds.), *The sourcebook on lesbian/gay health care* (2nd ed., pp. 151-161). Washington, DC: National Lesbian/Gay Health Foundation.

Ficarrotto, T. J. (1990). Racism, sexism, and erotophobia: Attitudes of heterosexuals toward homosexuals. *Journal of Homosexuality, 19*(1), 111-116.

Finnegan, D. G., & McNally, E. B. (1988). The lonely journey: Lesbians and gay men who are co-dependent. In M. Shernoff & W. A. Scott (Eds.), *The sourcebook on lesbian/gay health care* (2nd ed., pp. 173-179). Washington, DC: National Lesbian/Gay Health Foundation.

Freedman, M. (1967). *Homosexuality among women and psychological adjustment.* Unpublished doctoral dissertation, Case Western Reserve University, Cleveland.

Friend, R. A. (1989). Older lesbian and gay people: Responding to homophobia. *Marriage and Family Review, 14*(3/4), 241-263.

Gagnon, J. H., & Simon, W. (1973). *Sexual conduct.* Chicago: Aldine.

Galassi, F. S. (1991). A life-review workshop for gay and lesbian elders. *Journal of Gerontological Social Work, 16*(1/2), 75-86.

Garnets, L., Hancock, K. A., Cochran, S. D., Goodchilds, J., & Peplau, L. A. (1991). Issues in psychotherapy with lesbians and gay men. *American Psychologist, 46*(9), 964-972.

Gibbs, E. D. (1989). Psychosocial development of children raised by lesbian mothers: A review of research. *Women & Therapy, 8*(1/2), 65-75.

Glaus, K. H. (1989). Alcoholism, chemical dependency, and the lesbian client. *Women & Therapy, 8*(1/2), 131-144.

Gottman, J. S. (1989). Children of gay and lesbian parents. *Marriage and Family Review, 14*(3/4), 177-196.

Greene, B. A. (1986). When the therapist is white and the patient is black: Considerations for psychotherapy in the feminist heterosexual and lesbian communities. *Women & Therapy, 5*(2/3), 41-65.

Gundlach, R. H. (1967). Research project report. *The Ladder, 11,* 2-9.

Gundlach, R. H., & Riess, B. F. (1967). Birth order and sex of siblings in a sample of lesbians and non-lesbians. *Psychological Reports, 20,* 61-62.

Hassell, A., & Smith, E. W. (1975). Female homosexuals' concept of self, men, and women. *Journal of Personality Assessment, 42,* 83-90.

Hersch, P. (1991, January-February). Secret lives. *Networker,* 37-43.

Hetherington, C., & Orzek, A. (1989). Career counseling and life planning with lesbian women. *Journal of Counseling and Development, 68*(1), 52-57.

Hetrick, E. S., & Martin, A. D. (1987). Developmental issues and their resolution for gay and lesbian adolescents. *Journal of Homosexuality, 14*(1/2), 25-43.

Hidalgo, H., Peterson, T. L., & Woodman, N. J. (Eds.). (1985). *Lesbian and gay issues: A resource manual for social workers.* Silver Spring, MD: National Association of Social Workers.

Hooks, B. (1988, Summer). Reflections on homophobia and black communities. *Out/look*, pp. 22-25.

Hopkins, J. H. (1969). The lesbian personality. *British Journal of Psychiatry, 115*, 1433-1436.

Kahn, M. J. (1991). Factors affecting the coming out process for lesbians. *Journal of Homosexuality, 21*(3), 47-70.

Kanuha, V. (1990). Compounding triple jeopardy: Battering in lesbian of color relationships. *Women & Therapy, 9*(1/2), 169-184.

Kay, H. E., Soll, B., Clare, J., Eleston, M. R., Gershwin, B. S., Gershwin, P., Kogan, L. S., Torda, C., & Wilbur, C. B. (1967). Homosexuality in women. *Archives of General Psychiatry, 17*(5), 626-634.

Kehoe, M. (1988). Lesbians over sixty speak for themselves [Special issue]. *Journal of Homosexuality, 16*(3/4).

Kenyon, F. E. (1968). Studies in female homosexuality: Psychological test results. *Journal of Consulting Clinical Psychology, 32*, 510-513.

Kenyon, F. E. (1969). Studies in female homosexuality IV: Social and psychiatric aspects. *British Journal of Psychiatry, 114*, 1337-1350.

Kinsey, A. C., Pomeroy, W., & Martin, C. (1948). *Sexual behavior in the human male.* Philadelphia: W. B. Saunders.

Kinsey, A. C., Pomeroy, W., Martin, C., & Gebhard, P. H. (1953). *Sexual behavior in the human female.* Philadelphia: W. B. Saunders.

Klein, F., Sepekoff, B., & Wolf, T. (1985). Sexual orientation: A multi-variable dynamic process. *Journal of Homosexuality, 11*(1/2), 35-49.

Kus, R. J. (1990). *Keys to caring: Assisting your gay and lesbian clients.* Boston: Alyson.

LeVay, S. (1991). A difference in hypothalamic structure between heterosexual and homosexual men. *Science, 253*, 1034-1037.

Levy, E. (1992, January). Strengthening the coping resources of lesbian families. *Journal of Contemporary Human Services*, 23-31.

Lewis, L. A. (1984). The coming-out process for lesbians: Integrating a stable identity. *Social Work, 29*(5), 464-469.

Lewis, M. I. (1980). The history of female sexuality in the United States. In M. Kirkpatrick (Ed.), *Women's sexual development* (pp. 19-38). New York: Plenum Press.

Loiacano, D. K. (1989). Gay identity among black Americans: Racism, homophobia, and the need for validation. *Journal of Counseling and Development, 68*(1), 21-25.

Lott-Whitehead, L., & Tully, C. T. (1993). The families of lesbian mothers. *Smith College Studies in Social Work, 63*, 265-280.

Lukes, C. A., & Land, H. (1990). Biculturality and homosexuality. *Social Work, 35*(2), 155-161.

Markowitz, L. M. (1991, January-February). Homosexuality: Are we still in the dark? *Networker*, 27-35.

Martin, D. (Ed.). (1960). Some comparisons between male and female homosexuals [Special issue]. *The Ladder, 4*(12).

McDermott, D., Tyndall, L., & Lichtenberg, J. W. (1989). Factors related to counselor preference among gays and lesbians. *Journal of Counseling and Development, 68*(1), 31-35.

Mendola, M. (1980). *The Mendola report: A new look at gay couples.* New York: Crown.

Miranda, J., & Storms, M. (1989). Psychological adjustment of lesbians and gay men. *Journal of Counseling and Development, 68*(1), 41-45.

Modrcin, M. J., & Wyers, N. L. (1990). Lesbian and gay couples: Where they turn when help is needed. *Journal of Gay & Lesbian Psychotherapy, 1*(3), 89-104.

Morales, E. S. (1989). Ethnic minority families and minority gays and lesbians. *Marriage and Family Review, 14*(3/4), 217-239.

Morrow, S. L., & Hawxhurst, D. M. (1989). Lesbian partner abuse: Implications for therapists. *Journal of Counseling and Development, 68*(1), 58-62.

Murphy, B. C. (1989). Lesbian couples and their parents: The effects of perceived parental attitudes on the couple. *Journal of Counseling and Development, 68*(1), 46-51.

National Opinion Research Center (1989-1992). *General social survey.* University of Chicago: Author.

Ohlson, E. L., & Wilson, M. (1974). Differentiating female homosexuals from female heterosexuals by use of the MMPI. *Journal of Sex Research, 10*, 308-315.

Orzek, A. M. (1988). The lesbian victim of sexual assault: Special considerations for the mental health professional. *Women & Therapy, 8*(1/2), 107-117.

Ponse, B. (1978). *Identities in the lesbian world.* Westport, CT: Greenwood Press.

Poole, K. (1970). *A sociological approach to the etiology of female homosexuality and the lesbian social scene.* Unpublished doctoral dissertation, University of Southern California, Los Angeles.

Poor, M. (1982). Older lesbians. In M. Cruikshank (Ed.), *Lesbian studies: Present and future* (pp. 165-173). New York: Feminist Press.

Post, L. L. (1991). On remaining a radical lesbian feminist while training in psychiatry. *Women & Therapy, 11*(1), 91-102.

Reiter, L. (1989). Sexual orientation, sexual identity, and the question of choice. *Clinical Social Work Journal, 17*(2), 138-150.

Ritter, K. Y., & O'Neill, C. W. (1989). Moving through loss: The spiritual journey of gay men and lesbians. *Journal of Counseling and Development, 68*, 9-15.

Robinson, K. E. (1991). Gay youth support groups: An opportunity for social work intervention. *Social Work, 36*(5), 458-459.

Rofes, E. E. (1983). Lesbian and gay youth and suicide. In E. E. Rofes, *"I thought people like that killed themselves": Lesbians, gay men, and suicide* (pp. 34-48). San Francisco: Grey Fox.

Rogers, P. (1993, February 15). How many gays are there? *Newsweek,* p. 46.

Rothblum, E. D. (1988). Introduction: Lesbianism as a model of a positive lifestyle for women. *Women & Therapy, 8*(1/2), 1-12.

Rothblum, E. D. (1990). Depression among lesbians: An invisible and unresearchable phenomenon. *Journal of Gay & Lesbian Psychotherapy, 1*(3), 67-87.

Saghir, M. F., & Robins, E. (1969). Sexual behavior in the female homosexual. *Archives of General Psychiatry, 2,* 147-154.

Saunders, J. M., & Valente, S. M. (1987). Suicide risk among gay men and lesbians: A review. *Death Studies, 11*(1), 1-23.

Savin-Williams, R. C. (1989a). Gay and lesbian adolescents. *Marriage and Family Review, 14*(3/4), 197-216.

Savin-Williams, R. C. (1989b). Parental influences on the self-esteem in gay and lesbian youths: A reflected appraisals model. *Journal of Homosexuality, 17*(1/2), 93-109.

Schneider, M. (1989). Sappho was a right-on adolescent: Growing up lesbian. *Journal of Homosexuality, 17*(1/2), 111-130.

Schwartz, R. D. (1988). When the therapist is gay: Personal and clinical reflections. *Journal of Gay & Lesbian Psychotherapy, 1*(1), 41-50.

Seigel, R. J. (1987). Beyond homophobia: Learning to work with lesbian clients. *Women & Therapy, 6*(1/2), 125-133.

Shernoff, M., & Scott, W. A. (Eds.). (1988). *The sourcebook on lesbian/gay health care* (2nd Ed.). Washington, DC: National Lesbian/Gay Health Foundation.

Siegelman, M. (1972). Adjustment of homosexual and heterosexual women. *British Journal of Psychiatry, 120,* 477-481.

Siegelman, M. (1974). Parental behavior of homosexual and heterosexual women. *British Journal of Psychiatry, 124,* 14-21.

Smalley, S. (1987). Dependency issues in lesbian relationships. *Journal of Homosexuality, 14*(1/2), 125-135.

Smith, J. (1988). Psychopathology, homosexuality, and homophobia. *Journal of Homosexuality, 15*(1/2), 59-73.

Sobocinski, M. R. (1990). Ethical principles in the counseling of gay and lesbian adolescents: Issues of autonomy, competence, and confidentiality. *Professional Psychology: Research and Practice, 21*(4), 240-247.

Sophie, J. (1985/1986). A critical examination of stage theories of lesbian identity development. *Journal of Homosexuality, 12*(2), 39-51.

Sorella, N. (1991-1992). Lies, lies, and more lies. *Sinister Wisdom, 45,* 58-71.

Stein, T. S. (1983). Theoretical considerations in psychotherapy with gay men and lesbians. *Journal of Homosexuality, 15*(1/2), 75-95.

Strommen, E. F. (1989). "You're what?": Family member reactions to the disclosure of homosexuality. *Journal of Homosexuality, 18*(1/2), 37-58.

Swanson, D. W., Loomis, S. D., Lukesh, R., Cornin, R., & Smith, J. A. (1972). Clinical features of the female homosexual patient: A comparison with the heterosexual patient. *Journal of Nervous and Mental Disease, 155*(2), 119-124.

Tanner, D. M. (1978). *The lesbian couple.* Lexington, MA: D. C. Heath.

Thompson, N. L. (1971). *Family background and sexual identity in male and female homosexuals.* Unpublished doctoral dissertation, Emory University, Atlanta.

Thompson, N. L., McCandless, B. R., & Strickland, B. R. (1971). Personal adjustment of male and female homosexuals and heterosexuals. *Journal of Abnormal Psychology, 78,* 237-240.

Tripp, C. A. (1976). *The homosexual matrix.* New York: Signet.

Tully, C. T. (1983). *Social support systems of a selected sample of older women.* Unpublished doctoral dissertation, Virginia Commonwealth University, Richmond.

Tully, C. T. (1989). Caregiving: What do midlife lesbians view as important? *Journal of Gay & Lesbian Psychotherapy, 1*(1), 87-103.

Turner, P. H., Scadden, L., & Harris, M. B. (1990). Parenting in gay and lesbian families. *Journal of Gay & Lesbian Psychotherapy, 1*(3), 55-66.

Weinberg, G. (1973). *Society and the healthy homosexual.* New York: Anchor Books.

Wertheimer, D. M. (1990). Treatment and service interventions for lesbian and gay male crime victims. *Journal of Interpersonal Violence, 5*(3), 384-399.

Wilson, M. L., & Greene, R. L. (1971). Personality characteristics of female homosexuals. *Psychological Reports, 28,* 407-412.

Woodman, N. J. (1988). Mental health issues of relevance to lesbian women and gay men. *Journal of Gay & Lesbian Psychotherapy, 1*(1), 53-63.

Woodman, N. J. (Ed.). (1992). *Lesbian and gay lifestyles: A guide for counseling and education.* New York: Irvington.

Wyers, N. L. (1987). Homosexuality in the family: Lesbian and gay spouses. *Social Work, 32*(2), 143-148.

Potential Use of Single-System Designs for Evaluating Affirmative Psychotherapy with Lesbian Women and Gay Men

Ann E. MacEachron

SUMMARY. The paradigm shift from oppressive to affirmative psychotherapy for lesbian women and gay men is well under way in the clinical world. The challenge for both practitioners and researchers is to guide the development of affirmative models by evaluating their effectiveness. In this article, the author discusses the potential utility of single-system designs in terms of their methodological advantages in clinical research and their fit with affirmative practice.

The emphasis of lesbian and gay-affirmative psychotherapy models is to "value diversity and the integrity of each individual" (Morin & Charles, 1983, p. 334) by affirming the legitimacy of lesbian and gay lifestyles (Herek, Kimmel, Amaro, & Melton, 1991). Woodman and Lenna (1980), for example, discussed this process in terms of self-actualization where the self, to establish a definition of sexual orientation and to find affirmation of the "integrated self" through the acceptance of others, mediates between "inner needs and a supportive environment" (pp. 12-13). The func-

Ann E. MacEachron, PhD, is Professor at the School of Social Work, Arizona State University, Tempe, AZ 85287.

[Haworth co-indexing entry note]: "Potential Use of Single-System Designs for Evaluating Affirmative Psychotherapy with Lesbian Women and Gay Men." MacEachron, Ann E. Co-published simultaneously in *Journal of Gay & Lesbian Social Services* (The Haworth Press, Inc.) Vol. 3, No. 1, 1995, pp. 19-27; and: *Lesbian Social Services: Research Issues* (ed: Carol T. Tully) The Haworth Press, Inc., 1995, pp. 19-27; and: *Lesbian Social Services: Research Issues* (ed: Carol T. Tully) Harrington Park Press, an imprint of The Haworth Press, Inc., 1995, pp. 19-27. Multiple copies of this article/chapter may be purchased from The Haworth Document Delivery Center [1-800-3-HAWORTH; 9:00 a.m. - 5:00 p.m. (EST)].

19

tion of therapy "is to help the client eliminate the negative stereotypes that impede self-actualization and move toward a positive identity . . . [through] therapeutic acceptance and knowledgeable understanding" (pp. 12-13).

This article focuses on practitioner-based research that may guide the development of, and provide an empirical foundation for, affirmative models of psychotherapy with lesbian women and gay men. Of particular interest in this regard are single-system, single-subject, or N = 1 designs, which are a "special case of time series research using multiple-intervention design to control the time threats to internal validity" (Dooley, 1990, p. 246). Barlow, Hayes, and Nelsen (1984) placed single-system designs in the intermediate power range for establishing internal validity since case studies, percent of success studies and nonfactorial designs with control groups are less powerful, and factorial designs with control groups are more powerful but also more difficult. The advantage of single-system designs is that they provide relatively powerful, straightforward ways for practitioners to document client progress while concurrently evaluating the efficacy of therapeutic practices.

NEED FOR PRACTITIONER-BASED RESEARCH

Groups of people who have been and continue to be oppressed and discriminated against are particularly vulnerable to stereotyping and other negative misinformation. The foundation of such misinformation is heterosexism, racism, ethnocentrism, ageism, sexism, handicappism, or all of these. Correspondingly, individuals who are members of oppressed groups may also believe or internalize negative stereotypes about their group and thereby suffer a dual oppression from self and others. An important way to expose stereotypic misinformation and oppressive myths is to provide evidence that validates the uniqueness and humanity of each individual. Yet it seems a rule that the amount of available affirmative research is inversely proportional to the extent of societal oppression toward a group of people.

In terms of lesbian women and gay men, it probably is not surprising that psychotherapy and research have been and may still be biased, discriminatory, and exclusionary. One only needs to remember in this regard that the purpose of therapy has often been "to cure" the "psychopathology" of homosexuality and that most past research has focused on the diagnosis of homosexuality from the perspective of sickness models, early childhood causes of homosexuality, or the potential to change sexual orientation (Brooks, 1992; Falco, 1991; Herek et al., 1991). Indeed, the dominance of heterosexist bias in psychological research has been so vast that the American Psychological Association (APA) Task Force on Non-Homophobic Research recently listed 24 ways in which heterosexist bias may enter each stage of the research process, from formulating the research question to interpreting the results (Herek et al., 1991).

Given the emergence of affirmative models of psychotherapy with lesbian women and gay men (Falco, 1991; Garnets, Hancock, Cochran, Goodchilds, & Peplau, 1991; Morin & Charles, 1983; Woodman & Lenna, 1980), the time seems appropriate to provide an empirical and scientific foundation to evaluating lesbian and gay-affirmative psychotherapy. Moreover, with one exception, even the extent to which affirmative models have been adopted by practitioners is relatively unknown. A recent survey of 2,544 psychologists by the APA's Committee on Lesbian and Gay Concerns indicated only that there was variability among psychologists' self-reports of affirmatory practice with lesbians and gay men (Garnets et al., 1991). The authors' content analysis of these self-reports distinguished between psychological practice that was "biased, inadequate, or inappropriate" (p. 966) and practice that was "exemplary" (p. 968) in the areas of assessment, intervention, identity, relationships, therapist expertise, and therapist education.

The relative paucity of clinical research on these issues and the great need for lesbian and gay-affirmative research in general is unlikely to be well met unless practitioners working with lesbian and gay clients become involved. Practitioner involvement in efforts to define and improve methods for effective lesbian and gay-affirmative psychotherapy may be defined in many ways including theory and methods development, instruction, research dissemination, and clinical research.

RATIONALE FOR USING SINGLE-SYSTEM DESIGNS

Although there is an array of survey, experimental, and quasi-experimental designs from which to choose, single-system designs are inevitably and frequently recommended for practitioners to evaluate their practice (Barlow et al., 1984; Campbell, 1988; Edgington, 1987; Rosen, 1983). Single-system designs include using a subject as his/her own control; objectively measuring a subject's behavior, cognitive, or other outcomes of interest through standardized tests, checklists, or observation protocols; repeatedly measuring these behaviors over regular time intervals; and providing one or more well-specified interventions at predetermined times.

The effectiveness or ineffectiveness of the intervention is typically evaluated by a visual comparison of the subject's changes in behavior over time while undergoing intervention or while not receiving treatment (during the baseline before treatment, after the withdrawal of treatment, or both). The comparison of a subject's behaviors over time may show substantial change associated with the intervention, spontaneous improvement without intervention, no improvement, or may not provide any clear interpretation at all. Depending on the type of variation observed, practitioners may include additional interventions to understand client behavior in relation to each associated intervention. In this regard, Barlow et al. (1984) recommended using response-guided addition of interventions to understand and predict the patterns of variability highlighted by repeated measurement.

Single-system designs are recommended as a means to evaluate lesbian and gay-affirmative psychotherapy for a number of reasons. The first reason is that practitioners and single-system designs share a common focus on "single systems" such as an individual, a common goal of facilitating change within the single client system, and a common belief that developmental processes and change may differ for each client system even though there is an overarching developmental pattern across individuals.

Given this first reason, from a lesbian and gay-affirmative perspective, several associated advantages in using single-system designs exist. The confidentiality and privacy of the client system may be more easily safeguarded when single-system designs are used because there is only one subject involved. Issues of confidentiality are extremely important for lesbian and gay clients who, because of societal oppression, may believe that they must keep their sexual orientation hidden to preserve their jobs, family, or friends (Falco, 1991; Woodman & Lenna, 1980). At the same time, single-system designs emphasize the uniqueness of each individual. This emphasis on uniqueness, communicated through a discussion of research design with the client, may in itself help to contradict oppressive stereotypes of lesbian women and gay men.

Moreover, single-system designs are well-suited for exploring developmental pathways (Ottenbacher, Johnson, & Hojem, 1988) and as such may prove useful in understanding the multiple developmental pathways of lesbian and gay identity over time (Falco, 1991; Woodman & Lenna, 1980). The issue of selecting appropriate control groups has been especially problematic in research on lesbian women and gay men (Brooks, 1992; Herek et al., 1991). But by choosing a single-system design, this issue is avoided because the individual serves as his/her own control group (Barlow et al., 1984). Furthermore, lesbian and gay-affirmative psychotherapy emphasizes the potential need for intervention in group, family, organization, and community systems. A practitioner may well determine that the treatment plan should include group therapy, family therapy, or social advocacy because "gayness is a social identity that requires appropriate supportive environments for validation" (Woodman & Lenna, 1980, p. 110). Single-system designs are again appropriate, and indeed are often used, for evaluating change efforts at these other levels of intervention.

A second reason that single-system designs are often recommended to practitioners is because they are relatively easy to learn about from introductory research textbooks (Dooley, 1990; Nelsen, 1988; Rubin & Babbie, 1989; Royse, 1991). The ease of learning facilitates practitioner use of these designs to evaluate his or her practice without the necessity of undergoing a steep or prolonged learning curve.

A third reason is that although single-subject designs are easy to use and the results may be interpreted by visual inspection alone without statistical analysis, they also may be implemented with substantial elegance and sophistication in design (Barlow et al.,

1984; Edgington, 1987) and statistical analysis (Busk & Marascuilo, 1988; Gibson & Ottenbacher, 1988; Hilliker & Thyer, 1985; Ottenbacher, 1986; Ottenbacher, 1990a & 1990b; Ottenbacher, Johnson, & Hojem, 1988; Sharpley & Alavosius, 1988). Both simple and complex practice questions, therefore, may be entertained in the research process with this type of design (Bass, 1987).

A fourth reason single-subject designs are recommended is that most practitioners are eclectic in their use of intervention methods, including those who practice lesbian and gay-affirmative psychotherapies, which, by definition are eclectic. Single-system research design principles, such as the Barlow et al. (1984) response-guided intervention, fit well with eclectic approaches and thus are less likely to be intrusive or interfere with the psychotherapeutic process.

A fundamental issue in the use of single-system designs is how the findings on one subject may be generalized to any extent to another client as well as to different therapists or clinical settings. Bass's (1987) review of the philosophical, statistical, and sampling literature placed more importance on the number of replications than on the sample size of a study in determining generality. Bass's approach has also been adopted by others (Corcoran, 1985; Videka-Sherman, 1986; White, Rusch, Kazdin, & Hartmann, 1989) who have explored the technique of metaanalysis for aggregating data from single-system research. In this regard, practitioners of affirmative psychotherapy with lesbian women and gay men may wish to form collaborative research groups to replicate their individual results and thus enhance the generality of their findings. Such collaborative groups may not only provide collegial support for ongoing testing of the empirical validity of affirmative psychotherapy, but also may promote interest in affirmative psychotherapy and its effectiveness within broader professional communities.

CONCLUSION

It is each practitioner's ethical responsibility to be accountable for his or her practice and for generation of knowledge to improve practice. In this regard, a fundamental question that each practitioner must ultimately confront is: "Am I doing better than I could do by flipping pennies?" (Meehl, 1954, p. 136). Acceptance of this question leads inevitably to the necessity of becoming a "scientist-practitioner" who consumes new research findings, who evaluates the effectiveness of his/her practice interventions, and who disseminates research findings from his or her practice setting (Barlow et al., 1984, p. 4). This role set of expectations has been advocated in the ethical standards of social work and psychology for several decades. Moreover, clients not only accept, but prefer, conclusions based on single-system design outcomes to only receiving their practitioner's opinion on progress (Campbell, 1990).

Given the paradigm shift since the 1970s from oppressive and blaming to lesbian- and gay-affirmative psychotherapy, analytical research approaches that are supportive but also rigorous seem even more compulsory. It is not enough to support affirmative psychotherapy through verbal "shoulds," and it is not enough to "just" practice what you preach. As Herek et al. (1991) stated, "For the advancement of science and society, high-quality research is needed on a wide variety of issues related to sexual orientation" (p. 962). Without research, affirmative psychotherapy may be passed over as unsubstantiated beliefs or even propaganda. In contrast, rigorous research may advance the scope and depth of current affirmative models and may broaden their acceptance among professional communities. The challenge, then, is to select rigorous research methods such as single-system designs to establish an empirically valid foundation for affirmative psychotherapy with lesbian women and gay men.

REFERENCES

Barlow, D. H., Hayes, S. C., & Nelson, R. O. (1984). *The scientist practitioner: Research and accountability in clinical and educational settings.* New York: Pergamon Press.

Bass, R. F. (1987). The generality, analysis, and assessment of single-subject data. *Psychology in the Schools, 24*(2), 97-104.

Brooks, W. K. (1992). Research and the gay minority: Problems and possibilities. In N. J. Woodman (Ed.), *Lesbian and gay lifestyles: A guide for counseling and education* (pp. 201-215). New York: Irvington Publishers, Inc.

Busk, P. L., & Marascuilo, L. A. (1988). Autocorrelation in single-subject research: A counterargument to the myth of no autocorrelation. *Behavioral Assessment, 10*, 229-242.

Campbell, J. A. (1990). Ability of practitioners to estimate client acceptance of single-subject evaluation procedures. *Social Work, 35*, 9-14.

Campbell, P. H. (1988). Using a single-subject research design to evaluate the effectiveness of treatment. *American Journal of Occupational Therapy, 42*(11), 732-738.

Corcoran, K. J. (1985). Aggregating the idiographic data of single-subject design. *Social Work Research & Abstracts, 21*(2), 9-12.

Dooley, D. (1990). *Social research methods* (2nd ed.). Englewood Cliffs, NJ: Prentice-Hall.

Edgington, E. S. (1987). Randomized single-subject experiments and statistical tests. *Journal of Counseling Psychology, 34*(4), 437-442.

Falco, K. L. (1991). *Psychotherapy with lesbian clients: Theory into practice.* New York: Brunner/Mazel.

Garnets, L., Hancock, K. A., Cochran, S. D., Goodchilds, J., & Peplau, L. A. (1991). Issues in psychotherapy with lesbians and gay men. *American Psychologist, 46*(9), 964-972.

Gibson, G., & Ottenbacher, K. (1988). Characteristics influencing the visual analysis of single-subject data: An empirical analysis. *Journal of Applied Behavioral Science, 24*(3), 298-314.

Herek, G. M., Kimmel, D. C., Amaro, H., & Melton, G. B. (1991). Avoiding heterosexist bias in psychological research. *American Psychologist, 46*(9), 957-963.

Hilliker, G., & Thyer, B. A. (1985). Confidence intervals for statistical inference in single-subject research: A BASIC program. *Behavioral Engineering, 9*(3), 88-93.

Meehl, P. E. (1954). *Clinical vs. statistical prediction: A theoretical analysis and a review of the evidence.* Minneapolis, MN.: University of Minnesota Press.

Morin, S., & Charles, K. (1983). Heterosexual bias in psychotherapy. In J. Murray & P. R. Abramson (Eds.), *Bias in psychotherapy* (pp. 309-338). New York: Praeger.

Nelsen, J. C. (1988). Single-subject research. In R. M. Grinnell, Jr. (Ed.), *Social work research and evaluation* (3rd Ed.), (pp. 362-399). Itasca, IL: F. E. Peacock.

Ottenbacher, K. J. (1986). Reliability and accuracy of visually analyzing graphed data from single-subject designs. *American Journal of Occupational Therapy, 40*(7), 464-469.

Ottenbacher, K. J. (1990a). Visual inspection of single-subject data: An empirical analysis. *Mental Retardation, 28*(5), 283-290.

Ottenbacher, K. J. (1990b). When is a picture worth a thousand p values? A comparison of visual and quantitative methods to analyze single subject data. *Journal of Special Education, 23*(4), 436-449.

Ottenbacher, K. J., Johnson, M. B., & Hojem, M. (1988). The significance of clinical change and clinical change of significance: Issues and methods. *American Journal of Occupational Therapy, 42*(3), 156-163.

Rosen, A. (1983). Barriers to utilization of research by social work practitioners. *Journal of Social Service Research, 6*(3/4), 1-15.

Royse, D. (1991). *Research methods in social work.* Chicago: Nelson-Hall.

Rubin, A., & Babbie, E. (1989). *Research methods for social work.* Belmont, CA: Wadsworth.

Sharpley, C. F., & Alavosius, M. P. (1988). Autocorrelation in behavioral data: An alternative perspective. *Behavioral Assessment, 10,* 243-251.

Videka-Sherman, L. (1986). Alternative approaches to aggregating the results of single-subject studies. *Social Work Research & Abstracts, 22,* 22-23.

White, D. M., Rusch, F. R., Kazdin, A. E., & Hartmann, D. P. (1989). Applications of meta analysis in individual-subject research. *Behavioral Assessment, 11,* 281-296.

Woodman, N. J., & Lenna, H. R. (1980). *Counseling with gay men and women: A guide to facilitating positive life-styles.* San Francisco: Jossey-Bass.

Studying Partner Abuse
in Lesbian Relationships:
A Case for the Feminist Participatory
Research Model

Claire M. Renzetti

SUMMARY. Research on sensitive topics with a stigmatized and largely closeted population such as lesbians can be a daunting enterprise. Nevertheless, such research is valuable for revealing the serious social problems that lesbians experience, for documenting the extent of these problematic experiences, for uncovering the causes of the problems, and for suggesting solutions. In this article, the author argues that the methodological difficulties inherent in undertaking such research can often be best addressed by utilizing a feminist participatory research model. The benefits of this model, examined in the context of one researcher's experience in studying partner abuse in lesbian relationships, include allowing members of invisible and oppressed groups to shape research about themselves and to give voice to their experiences; allowing researchers to share their professional skills, but also become learners during the research process; improving the quality and accuracy of the data; and facilitating personal and social transformation (in the researcher as well as the researched).

Claire M. Renzetti, PhD, is Professor in the Department of Sociology, St. Joseph's University, Philadelphia, PA 19131.

[Haworth co-indexing entry note]: "Studying Partner Abuse in Lesbian Relationships: A Case for the Feminist Participatory Research Model." Renzetti, Claire M. Co-published simultaneously in *Journal of Gay & Lesbian Social Services* (The Haworth Press, Inc.) Vol. 3, No. 1, 1995, pp. 29-42; and: *Lesbian Social Services: Research Issues* (ed: Carol T. Tully) The Haworth Press, Inc., 1995, pp. 29-42; and: *Lesbian Social Services: Research Issues* (ed: Carol T. Tully) Harrington Park Press, an imprint of The Haworth Press, Inc., 1995, pp. 29-42. Multiple copies of this article/chapter may be purchased from The Haworth Document Delivery Center [1-800-3-HAWORTH; 9:00 a.m. - 5:00 p.m. (EST)].

The methodological difficulties in undertaking research on partner abuse in lesbian relationships seemed overwhelming at first. As
a social scientist schooled in traditional positivist standards of research, the author worried about the issues of sampling, study design, instrument construction, reactive effects, generalizability, and
so on. As a feminist social scientist, however, the author was also
aware of alternative methodologies, although less well versed in
them. This article is as much an autobiography of the author's
education in feminist methodology–an account of "learning by doing," if you will–as it is an evaluation of the utility of a particular
research model–the feminist participatory model–for conducting
research on sensitive topics with a stigmatized and largely closeted
population: lesbians.

In this article, the author compares the feminist participatory
model with the positivist model. She then discusses the application
of the feminist participatory model in the research on partner abuse
in lesbian relationships, highlighting the major benefits in such a
project. Furthermore, the author suggests ways in which a broad-
ened use of the feminist participatory model may improve research
on other aspects of lesbians' lives and intimate relationships.

THE FEMINIST CHALLENGE TO POSITIVIST HEGEMONY

Although there is no single, unified feminist methodology, several principles typically underlie feminist research that distinguish it
from traditional positivist research. Cancian (1992, pp. 626-627),
based on an earlier review by Cook and Fonow (1984), identified
five elements of feminist methodology: (1) a focus on gender and
gender inequality that, in turn, implies a strong political and moral
commitment to reducing inequality; (2) the goal of describing or
"giving voice" to people's (especially women's) personal, everyday experiences, particularly the experiences of marginalized
people; (3) action or policy implications with the goal of social
change to improve the conditions under which particular women
live; (4) a built-in reflexivity that critically examines "how the
research process is shaped by the gender, race, class, and sexual
orientation of the researcher, and by the broader social and cultural

context" (Cancian, 1992, p. 626); and (5) a rejection of the traditional relationship between researcher and "researched" in favor of methods that give research "subjects" more power in the research process (see also Reinharz, 1992).

Perhaps the most basic feature of feminist methodology is its recognition of gender as a central category of research. Traditional social sciences research, in contrast, typically has omitted an explicit examination of gender (e.g., by using all male samples, but generalizing the findings to all people) or has incorporated women as the "other" or the "exception" (e.g., by accepting as the norm men's characteristic ways of speaking or acting in particular situations). By including gender as a (often *the*) major component in a research project, feminist researchers have uncovered and documented widespread gender inequality. More recently, they have begun to consider the intersecting effects of multiple inequalities: sexism, racism, social class inequality, heterosexism, ageism, and ableism. Thus, as Cancian (1992), who referenced Hooks' (1984) research has pointed out, "Feminists have clarified how the concept of 'women in general' falsely universalizes and privileges the perspective of middle-class, heterosexual white women and denies and devalues the experiences of other women" (Cancian, 1992, p. 627).

At this point it should be clear to readers who received their original social sciences training within a positivist methodological framework, that the notion of value-free, completely objective research is an anathema to feminist social scientists. Indeed, one of the most significant contributions of feminist methodologists is their debunking of the myth of value-free scientific inquiry. Traditional positivist research, which claimed to be value free and objective, has been revealed as heavily laden with the values and biases of the researchers (white, male) who conducted it (Maguire, 1987; Reinharz, 1992). At the same time, however, feminist researchers, in rejecting the notion of value-free science, have not rejected "scientific standards" in their research. Rather, feminists simply have called for open acknowledgement by researchers of their assumptions, beliefs, sympathies, and biases. Feminists question not only the possibility, but also the desirability, of value-free social sciences. Hence, researchers must not only document inequality, but also commit themselves to reducing or eliminating it (Maguire, 1987).

Traditional positivist social science research also has been characterized by a rigid separation or detachment of the "knower" from the "known."

> The researcher is the expert who selects a problem for study, decides how it is to be studied, designs the research instruments, draws a sample, collects and analyzes the data, and presents the findings (usually just to professional colleagues) at conferences or in scholarly publications. Sometimes, but not often, researchers share their findings with those they have studied. Even then, however, this commonly takes the form of the researcher imparting upon them her or his "enlightened" view. In traditional social science, those studied are truly research subjects. (Renzetti, 1992, pp. 7-8)

In sociology, this approach has resulted in a strong bias toward random sampling strategies, survey methods, and quantitative analysis as the most rigorous and scientifically sound research techniques (Reinharz, 1992).

In contrast, feminist researchers reject the researcher/subjects dichotomy, seeing the research process instead as a collaborative enterprise. Both researcher and researched are involved in the project as humans. Researchers are encouraged to "start from their own experience"; to freely share with the researched information about themselves, their personal lives, and their opinions; and to adhere to a feminist ethic by complying with requests for help and offering advice and direct assistance (Cook and Fonow, 1984; Oakley, 1981; Reinharz, 1992). Rather than biasing data in a negative sense, feminists maintain that self-disclosure and the establishment of reciprocity between researcher and researched contributes to the success of a project (see, for example, Kennedy Bergen, 1993).

At the same time, feminists are committed to giving voice to people's personal, everyday experiences, particularly the experiences of those who have been marginalized in a society. This commitment has led to a strong bias in favor of convenience and purposive sampling strategies and qualitative methods, such as depth interviews, ethnographies, and life histories. Feminists, though, have not totally abandoned survey research and quantitative techniques; rather, to paraphrase Reinharz (1992, p. 76), the feminist response to survey research and quantitative analysis is best characterized as ambivalent. Feminists acknowledge that survey research can be valuable in documenting a problem that previously was thought to be uncommon or that was ignored altogether. Furthermore, they recognize the political and legal power of statistical presentations. Nevertheless, they are critical of a "statistical-industrial complex" (Reinharz, 1992; the source of this concept is Edith Altbach [1974], who apparently discovered the term in an essay written by Betty Gray [1971]). In addition, they are quick to point out how survey-based data and statistical analyses have been used against women and other marginalized groups by disguising particular problems, creating erroneous information that carries "statistical authority," and reinforcing stereotypes (Reinharz, 1992). Consequently, feminist researchers typically advocate the use of multiple methods in a research project, particularly if one of the methods is quantitative or survey based.

The rejection of the notion of the researcher as detached from the researched in favor of a model of research as a collaborative enterprise has led some feminist researchers to advocate the use of participatory methods. Maguire (1987), whose own work is an exemplar of the feminist participatory model, defines *participatory research* as combining three activities: (1) investigation, (2) education, and (3) action.

> It is a method of social *investigation* of problems, involving participation of oppressed and ordinary people in problem posing and solving. It is an *educational* process for the researcher and participants, who analyze the structural causes of named problems through collective discussion and interaction. Finally, it is a way for researchers and oppressed people to join in solidarity to take collective *action,* both short and long term, for radical social change. (p. 35; for other examples of the feminist participatory model, see Kleiber and Light, 1978; and Mies, 1983)

In this model, the research relationship is clearly reciprocal rather than hierarchical. The researcher, rather than being a detached expert, engages the participation of community members from the outset, recognizing that both parties bring to a project unique skills, knowledge, and resources. As Maguire (1987) put it, "We both know some things, neither of us knows everything. Working together we will both know more, and we will both learn more about how to know" (p. 40).

In feminist participatory research, the researched remain active participants throughout the project, identifying problems to be studied; contributing to the development of research instruments; analyzing and interpreting data; and, perhaps most important, deciding on the uses of the data. Recall that major goals of feminist methodology are challenging inequality and improving the life conditions of oppressed groups. Feminist participatory research calls for a research project to empower the researched to develop and implement strategies that address specific problems that concern them; these problems typically stem from their unequal and marginalized status in society.

Undoubtedly, the feminist participatory model poses a tall order for researchers, one that some may be reluctant to try to fill. However, this model is especially useful for research with lesbians who, as a group, are stigmatized and largely closeted. The results of such a project may be beneficial to the researcher, the researched, and to the social sciences and general communities as a whole.

STUDYING LESBIAN PARTNER ABUSE
USING A FEMINIST PARTICIPATORY FRAMEWORK

The current research on partner abuse in lesbian relationships would not have been possible without the use of the feminist participatory model. For one thing, as a heterosexual woman, the author is an outsider to the lesbian community. In addition, the author's position as a social scientist at a Roman Catholic university makes her more suspect. The topic was one that was not taken seriously by the heterosexual social scientific community. In addition, many in the lesbian community would have preferred to leave the topic undiscussed, given that it could tarnish the ideal image of lesbian relationships in the community and simultaneously draw attention to a problem that could further fuel already-rampant societal homophobia. The following describes how the feminist participatory model was used in the current project as well as its major benefits.

Origin of the Questionnaire

The project began in spring 1985, when the author contacted an activist at a local battered women's service agency in Philadelphia regarding an advertisement in a lesbian/gay newspaper for a community forum on lesbian battering. The author requested additional information about the problem of lesbian battering and also inquired whether the community might be interested in a research project on this problem. As a result of this initial contact, the activist provided a list of the limited resources available at the time on lesbian battering (most of which were articles in feminist/lesbian publications) and arranged a meeting between the author and activists in the lesbian community concerned with the problem of lesbian partner abuse. (Although the women who attended this meeting became the core group that worked on the research project, the group was not a closed circle. Input also was sought throughout the project from representatives from a battered women's group and members of the local lesbian community, several of whom were battered lesbians.)

It was immediately clear at the initial meeting that the activists and author each would bring to a research project different talents, skills, and knowledge. The author had access to funding sources, grant writing experience, and technical skills in research methodology and data analysis, but few contacts in the lesbian community. Moreover, the author knew far less about lesbian relationships than she originally presumed, and had no experience, either direct or indirect, with battered lesbians or lesbian batterers. The activists, in contrast, brought years of collective experience in the battered women's movement and experiential knowledge of lesbian relationships, of the lesbian community in their city and other parts of the country, and, most important, of lesbian battering. The activists and the author agreed that an empirical study of lesbian battering would be a significant step in "naming the violence" that some lesbians were suffering in their intimate relationships; in clarifying similarities and differences between battered lesbians and battered heterosexual women; and in identifying potential strategies to reduce or end the violence by raising community awareness about the problem, assisting victims, and holding batterers accountable. Nevertheless, a number of serious issues had to be addressed before any formal project planning could get underway; among these was the question of *ownership.*

The activists initially asked the question of who would own the project: The author? The activists? The funding source? A combination of the three? They were concerned with how a heterosexual social scientist might use the findings. The author was concerned that the findings, which would have broad implications for the study of domestic violence in general, be disseminated to other researchers studying abuse by intimates. All were concerned that the funding source–the university with which the author is affiliated–might ultimately try to control or censor the findings. (This fear eventually proved unfounded. The university administration and colleagues provided extensive support throughout the course of the project.) This was the first point at which the feminist participatory model came into play, because the model dictates that project ownership is joint. The resolution to the issue of ownership was that the author would take responsibility for disseminating the findings among academics, social services providers, and other practitioners; the activists would take responsibility for disseminating the findings within the lesbian community. Over time, however, these "boundaries" became obviously artificial, and the activists and the author frequently worked in the other's "territory."

The issue of ownership, however, was not settled at that first meeting. To a large extent, it evolved over the life span of the project, but all were clear from the outset that they were "in this together" and that the author could not claim sole ownership of what would be a collective/collaborative product. That decided, meetings were held at least once a week for several weeks and typically lasted two hours or longer as the group planned the project design and began to develop the research instruments.

Recruiting study volunteers would be difficult. Drawing a random sample would be impossible, but the author also was unwilling to adopt the approach used by a number of other researchers by simply distributing questionnaires at an event (such as a women's music festival) where there might be a large number of participants who would be lesbians. The resolution was again collaborative and drew on the group's respective skills and knowledge. The author suggested advertising for study participants; the activists suggested the medium. The group designed the ads and public announcements of the study, but the activists designed a brochure about lesbian partner abuse in which study announcements and self-mailing cards to request questionnaires were inserted. (The sampling strategy as well as the issue of sampling bias are discussed at length in Renzetti, 1992.)

Despite the feminist emphasis on qualitative methods, the group decided that a questionnaire would be the best way to at least begin to collect data. Given the sensitive nature of the topic, a questionnaire would provide study volunteers with anonymity and thus be less threatening than an interview. In addition, a questionnaire could potentially reach a larger number of women and perhaps could better gauge incidence and various demographic variables of interest.

After considerable discussion of the issues to cover in the research instrument, the author drafted a questionnaire and brought it to a meeting, confident that it would require only minor revisions before it would be ready for distribution. The first draft of the questionnaire, however, was subjected to intense scrutiny within the group, and an extensive dialogue ensued in which there were pointed disagreements–not only between the author and the activists but also among the activists–over virtually every item. Although the author shared her knowledge of scaling and other methodological technicalities, the activists patiently sensitized the author to issues of language and variations in experience. The questionnaire went through six drafts over a period of nine months. That may seem to some researchers like an inordinate amount of time for questionnaire development, but the quality of the end product is attested to by the number of respondents who wrote notes or told the author during subsequent interviews that completing the questionnaire actually contributed to their recovery from the trauma of their abuse experiences. Apparently, the research project was empowering for many of the study volunteers, a goal that is central to the feminist participatory model.

The twelve-page questionnaire on their relationships with abusive partners was distributed to more than 200 women who had responded to the ads. Of those women, 100 completed the questionnaire. Although the questionnaire provided a database, it had disadvantages. Most of the items were close-ended, offering a limited number of response categories. Although there were a few open-ended questions, it seemed unlikely that the instrument could adequately convey the complexity of the interactions and feelings the respondents were asked to describe. It was hardly surprising, then, that many respondents wrote in explanations of their answers beside the response categories they had circled. A number of women attached extra pages of detailed information to their completed questionnaires.

Interview

Like other feminist researchers, the activists and author wanted to give voice to these women's experiences. Consequently, on the last page of the questionnaire, respondents were asked if they would be interested in being interviewed. The interview was to be largely unstructured to provide the women with an opportunity to simply tell their stories and to highlight what they considered to be the most significant aspects of their battering experiences. Nevertheless, a preliminary review of the questionnaire data raised several issues that needed to be explored in greater detail in the interviews (e.g., respondents' explanations of why the battering had occurred, how the battering experience had affected respondents' subsequent intimate relationships, factors that inhibited or encouraged respondents to end the abusive relationships). The development of the interview schedule followed the same collaborative process as the development of the questionnaire. However, because the interview was to be largely unstructured and because of the group's experience in developing the questionnaire, it took considerably less time to develop the interview schedule, which went through only three revisions.

The author conducted all of the interviews, either in person or by phone, and each was tape recorded. Of the questionnaire respondents, 70 (70%) also volunteered to be interviewed. The interviewer consciously tried to break down any barriers between researcher and researched. The interviewer freely offered advice and emotional support during what were undoubtedly painful recountings of traumatic experiences; when possible and when asked, the interviewer made referrals to specific help providers, such as support groups for battered lesbians, that had been identified during the course of the project. The interviewer typically concluded the interview by asking the respondent if there was anything she wanted to know about the interviewer or if she would like to give any feedback on the project. This request contributed to the reciprocity of the research relationship and provided respondents with an opportunity to "talk back" to the researcher regarding the research (see Cook and Fonow, 1984; Kennedy Bergen, 1993).

Analysis

To preserve the confidentiality of study volunteers, the author coded all the questionnaire data and personally transcribed each taped interview. However, everyone in the group received copies of interview transcripts with all identifying information deleted and of computer printouts containing the aggregate data analysis. Interpretation of the data was undertaken collectively, although the group approached the task from different angles. The author applied her knowledge from an extensive review of the social sciences literature on domestic violence and, to a lesser extent, on lesbian relationships. The activists applied their experiential knowledge as counselors, advocates, and administrators in the battered women's movement and as partners in lesbian relationships, some as formerly battered lesbians. The author taught the activists how to read and interpret various statistical tests. Together the group discerned what the data meant and then undertook the task of explaining the findings to others.

Presentation of Findings

Before any of the findings were published or discussed in a public forum, the group prepared a report summarizing the questionnaire data for the study volunteers and distributed it to those for whom the group had mailing addresses. This effort represented a commitment to a feminist ethic of care for study volunteers. It also provided another opportunity for respondents to provide feedback on the research, as requested in the letter accompanying the report.

Moreover, it signified a commitment to the principle that the research should be empowering for the participants.

At this point, the group meetings became less frequent and a number of activists in the group dropped out for a variety of reasons. Nevertheless, as each member of the group pursued her own writing and education projects based on the research, a few members continued to meet periodically, if only to share new ideas or to comment on the written work or community activity. At least two members of the original group have reviewed nearly all of the author's written work on the project. Their comments and suggestions have formed the primary basis for subsequent revisions. This is not censorship; rather, it is evidence of ongoing collaboration. Specific details on the start of the project as well as study findings are discussed in the book, *Violent Betrayal: Partner Abuse in Lesbian Relationships* (Renzetti, 1992), where readers can better evaluate the "quality" of the project by whichever scientific standards they choose.

THE BROADER APPLICABILITY
OF THE FEMINIST PARTICIPATORY MODEL

The use of the feminist participatory model in the current study of partner abuse in lesbian relationships evolved during the course of the project; it was not something that either the author or the activists originally identified as their explicit research perspective. It emerged as the guiding framework for two reasons. First, each person involved in the planning and design of the study was committed to feminist principles of equality, partnership, and democratization. Second, the model simply made sense in terms of the goals for the project: to reveal the many dimensions of a problem that had been hidden and ignored, that is, to give voice to the experiences of battered lesbians; to identify strategies for solving this problem; and, especially, to empower battered lesbians, who have lived the consequences of this problem in their everyday lives.

In a way, then, the feminist participatory model chose the group; the group did not intentionally choose it at the outset. With hindsight, however, the broader utility of the model for research with lesbians is clear. As a stigmatized and, in many respects, invisible population, lesbians who participate in a collaborative research project benefit as both teachers and learners. Rather than having an analysis of their experiences imposed on them by "experts," who themselves may or may not be lesbians, lesbian research participants may shape the problems to be studied; how they are studied; and how research findings are interpreted, disseminated, and used. They may use the research findings themselves to bring about personal and social transformation.

At the same time, researchers also benefit as teachers and learners. They share their professional skills, but the participation of the researched in the project means that the study becomes truly an educational process for the researcher. This participation, in turn, improves the quality and accuracy of the research by ensuring that the most significant issues (from the perspectives of both researcher and researched) are identified and studied; that meaningful (in terms of the experiences of the researched) and nonalienating research instruments are developed; that the data collected are analyzed in the realistic context of the researched's everyday lives; and that the project has a practical impact in terms of personal and social transformation for the researcher as well as the researched.

Finally, the social sciences and general communities benefit in that knowledge is not created for knowledge's sake. Rather, in a feminist participatory research project, the knowledge created enriches practice and informs public policy making. In this sense, a feminist participatory research project is not completed until desired social changes are actualized. Both the researcher and the researched must make a strong, long-term commitment, but, ultimately, it may be worth it if the life conditions of oppressed and invisible groups are improved and social scientific inquiry becomes an essential element of social change.

REFERENCES

Altbach, E. H. (1974). *Women in America*. Lexington, MA: D. C. Heath.

Cancian, F. M. (1992). Feminist science: Methodologies that challenge inequality. *Gender and Society, 6*, 623-642.

Cook, J., & Fonow, M. (1984). Knowledge and women's interests: Issues of epistemology and methodology in feminist sociological research. *Sociological Inquiry, 56*, 2-29.

Gray, B. M. (1971, June 14). Economics of sex bias: The "diuse" of women. *The Nation*, pp. 742-744.

Hooks, B. (1984). *Feminist theory: From margin to center.* Boston: South End Press.

Kennedy Bergen, R. (1993). Interviewing survivors of marital rape: Doing feminist research on sensitive topics. In C. M. Renzetti & R. M. Lee (Eds.), *Researching sensitive topics* (pp. 197-211). Newbury Park, CA: Sage.

Kleiber, N., & Light, L. (1978). *Caring for ourselves: An alternative structure for health care.* Vancouver: University of British Columbia, School of Nursing.

Maguire, P. (1987). *Doing participatory research: A feminist approach.* Amherst, MA: The Center for International Education, University of Massachusetts at Amherst.

Mies, M. (1983). Towards a methodology of feminist research. In G. Bowles & R. Duelli-Klein (Eds.), *Theories of women's studies* (pp. 117-139). Boston: Routledge and Kegan Paul.

Oakley, A. (1981). Interviewing women: A contradiction in terms. In H. Roberts (Ed.), *Doing feminist research* (pp. 30-61). London: Routledge and Kegan Paul.

Reinharz, S. (1992). *Feminist methods in social research.* New York: Oxford University Press.

Renzetti, C. M. (1992). *Violent betrayal: Partner abuse in lesbian relationships.* Newbury Park, CA: Sage.

Methodological Issues in Research
on Older Lesbians

Sharon Jacobson

SUMMARY. Little attention has been paid to methodological issues in conducting research on older lesbians. Investigators who have conducted research in minority communities have also discussed this problem. In this article the author integrates these two bodies of literature. In addition, the author suggests that to address these concerns, future research on older lesbians should identify and examine older lesbians of color and should be designed so that the methodology is participatory in nature, places both the respondent and researcher on equal footing, is flexible so that it can adapt to existing group norms, and can be integrated into other research methods.

Methodological issues in the study of homosexuality have received minimal attention in the past. Leznoff (1956) and Warren (1977) addressed the concerns encountered by investigators who had conducted interviews and phenomenological research with gay males. Weinberg (1970) examined the differences and similarities between male homosexual samples. The existence of age and source sample deficiencies in studies of male homosexuals was discussed by Harry (1986). Bell (1975) identified the theoretical and conceptual deficiencies in research on male homosexuals. Ex-

Sharon Jacobson, MA, is a Doctoral Student at the Department of Recreation and Leisure Studies, University of Georgia, Athens, GA 30602-2303.

[Haworth co-indexing entry note]: "Methodological Issues in Research on Older Lesbians." Jacobson, Sharon. Co-published simultaneously in *Journal of Gay & Lesbian Social Services* (The Haworth Press, Inc.) Vol. 3, No. 1, 1995, pp. 43-56; and: *Lesbian Social Services: Research Issues* (ed: Carol T. Tully) The Haworth Press, Inc., 1995, pp. 43-56; and: *Lesbian Social Services: Research Issues* (ed: Carol T. Tully) Harrington Park Press, an imprint of The Haworth Press, Inc., 1995, pp. 43-56. Multiple copies of this article/chapter may be purchased from The Haworth Document Delivery Center [1-800-3-HAWORTH; 9:00 a.m. - 5:00 p.m. (EST)].

isting research on older lesbians has delineated methodological limitations and weaknesses of such research, yet has overlooked a general discussion of these issues.

First, this article presents the common methodological issues regarding sample representativeness in studies involving older lesbians. Second, the author discusses methodological issues that have been identified by researchers of other minorities. Third, the author examines these methodological issues and offers implications for future research involving older lesbians.

SAMPLE REPRESENTATIVENESS

Throughout the research on older lesbians several methodological issues have emerged that focused on sample representativeness. Those issues include definition of the population, enumeration of the population, lack of ethnic/racial representation, urban bias, and awareness of organizations and resources.

Definition of the Population

Barrett (1989) raised an interesting question when asking, "But who is a lesbian?" (p. 19). The lack of a clearly delineated definition of lesbianism conceptually prohibits a sample from being representative (Berger, 1984). Self-identification as a lesbian or participation in a lesbian organization have been the most commonly used methods of identifying sample members (Berger, 1984; Chafetz, Sampson, Beck, & West, 1974; Galassi, 1991; Kehoe, 1986, 1988; Lucco, 1987; Minnigerode & Adelman, 1978; Riege-Laner, 1979; Tully, 1989). Historically, a *lesbian* has been defined as "a woman whose primary erotic, psychological, emotional and social interest is in a member of her own sex, even though that interest may not be overtly expressed" (Martin & Lyon, 1972). However, as Poor (1982) clearly pointed out, older women may be reluctant to identify or label themselves as lesbians. This attitude was reflected in Kehoe (1988) by two respondents. In response to the question, "What word do you prefer to use to describe your emotional and/or sexual preference?" (p. 46), one woman responded "Anything, but lesbian" (p. 46). Another woman responded, "I think I would not like to be identified by sexual preference–either as a homosexual or a heterosexual" (p. 47). Of the women who participated in Tully's (1989) study of caregiving, 92% ($n = 67$) indicated that they were not completely open about their sexual orientation. Furthermore, there are women commonly called "lace curtain lesbians" (Cruik-shank, 1990, p. 81) whose primary interests may be in relationships with other women, yet they choose not to identify themselves as lesbians. In this article, the definition offered by Martin and Lyon (1972) is adopted for both women who self-identify as lesbians and those who choose not to.

Enumeration of the Older Lesbian

How many elderly lesbians exist in the United States? Numerous estimates have been offered about the size of the lesbian population in general and specifically about older lesbians. One factor in determining the estimated number of older lesbians is agreement on the bottom age to be used in conducting research on older lesbians. Lucco (1987) in a review of six studies on older lesbians reported a range in bottom ages from 40 to 60 years. Wolf (1978) used a bottom age of 40 years to match the age of the youngest possible member of the organization. Kehoe (1986) used a bottom age of 65 years.

Kinsey, Pomeroy, and Martin (1953) estimated that approximately 6% of the female population in the United States is lesbian. Poor (1982) estimated that, in 1977, a minimum of 834,000 lesbians older than age 65 years were living in the United States. In 1989, using the same estimate of 6%, a minimum of 1,100,880 lesbians older than age of 65 years were living in this country (U.S. Department of Commerce, 1991).

Ethnic/Racial Representation

Estimates indicate that 25% of the general U. S. population comprises ethnic/racial minorities other than Caucasian (Morales, 1990). However, despite researchers' efforts to recruit women of various ethnic/racial minorities, the samples in the majority of studies of older lesbians have included only white respondents (Adelman, 1990; Berger, 1984; Kehoe, 1986). Other studies have not reported on the ethnic/racial backgrounds of their participants (Galassi, 1991; Lucco, 1987; Minnigerode & Adelman, 1978). Those studies that have included women of ethnic/racial minorities in their samples have experienced low response rates. Barrett (1989) reported that, of 125 women interviewed, only 10% ($n = 13$) were women of ethnic/racial minorities. Kehoe (1988) reported that of 100 women who responded to her study of lesbians older than age 60 years, only 7 were of minority ethnic or racial backgrounds. Of the 73 women who participated in Tully's (1989) study, 96% ($n = 70$) were white, whereas only 4% ($n = 3$) of the respondents were Hispanic.

Urban Bias

Another issue in the area of sample representativeness is the focus of attention on urban areas that offer lesbian organizations, publications, and services geared to meet the age-specific needs of older lesbians. Numerous studies on older lesbians have focused their recruitment efforts on urban areas (Adelman, 1990; Berger, 1984; Minnigerode & Adelman, 1978; Raphael & Robinson, 1984). Although use of these areas facilitates the identification and recruitment of sample members within one setting, it fails to consider older lesbians who reside in nonurban settings. Kehoe's (1988) study indicated a need for attention to be paid to the nonurban settings. Of the 100 women who responded to Kehoe's (1988) study, 44% of the women were from urban settings and 56% were from rural, suburban, or small towns.

Awareness of Organizations and Resources

The bias towards older women who avail themselves of support organizations and publications (Berger, 1984) is another issue regarding sample representativeness. Although involvement in lesbian organizations may facilitate participation in a study, participants may not represent older lesbians in general. Berger (1982) reported that older lesbians typically made minimal use of lesbian support organizations and instead preferred to find support in a private network of friends.

METHODOLOGICAL ISSUES ON RESEARCH WITH MINORITIES

The literature on conducting research with ethnic/racial minorities raises several concerns that have not been discussed in the literature on lesbians and aging. Montero (1977), through an examination of articles that appeared in a special issue of the *Journal of Social Issues,* identified several themes that were consistent in the literature on research in minority communities. These themes included theoretical concerns; ethical concerns; problems in gaining access; survey methodology and field research; issues of design; and issues of measurement.

Theoretical Concerns

Numerous studies have reported on and fully discussed the theoretical and conceptual problems in conducting research on ethnic/racial minorities. The theoretical concerns identified throughout the literature focus on three issues: (1) the generalizability of existent theoretical orientations and conceptual frameworks to ethnic/racial minorities, (2) the confusion that stems from stereotyping the nature of ethnic/racial minority cultures, and (3) the oppressive and negative focus of research on ethnic/racial minorities.

The first concern revolves around the need to be sensitive to the development and formulation of theoretical frameworks that apply to ethnic/racial minorities (Warren, 1977). Numerous theoretical frameworks exist that have been formulated and tested on samples of primarily white males. The application of theoretical orientations and conceptual frameworks that have been imposed from outsider populations lends itself to the distortion of research (Zinn, 1979).

The second concern stems from the generalizability of cultures. Mindel and Kail (1989) discussed the tendency by nonminority researchers to make generalizations about ethnic/racial minority cultures. They stated that "there is often an oversimplified notion of the monolithic nature of [a] group's culture" (p. 194). It is important to recognize the differences within a culture as well as between the cultures. This concept has been applied to research on gender as well (Henderson, Bialeschki, Shaw, & Freysinger, 1989).

The third concern stems from the oppressive and negative focus of social issues research on ethnic/racial minorities. Social scientists have concentrated their research efforts on "the minorities, the institutionalized, the disadvantaged, and the stigmatized" (Warren, 1977, p. 94). Mindel and Kail (1989) argued that the focus of research has revolved around negative aspects of the lives of these individuals and has not examined the social structures that have contributed to the oppression of these populations. The tendency to place the blame and responsibility for the quality of one's life is widespread. The failure to account for historical, political, and social influences may demonstrate not only a negative attitude toward the group studied but a lack of understanding of the culture itself (Mindel & Kail, 1989).

Ethical Concerns

Methodologists who have conducted social research on minority communities have encountered numerous ethical concerns. Among these concerns is the issue of exploitation of minority groups by researchers (Kahana & Felton, 1977; Montero, 1977; Weiss, 1977; Zinn, 1979). Minority communities have perceived that researchers exploit subjects' economic and social conditions to enhance their own careers through the presentation of papers, securing of grants, and publication of books and journal articles (Weiss, 1977). In some minority communities, this feeling of exploitation has led to mistrust for researchers regardless of ethnicity (Zinn, 1979). This situation has prompted researchers to develop relationships with minority communities that foster trust and respect (Weiss, 1977).

Exploitation and stigmatization have served as a double-edged sword for those who have selected to research homosexual communities or other stigmatized groups. The perception of the researcher outside of that role might not only impact the development of relationships with informants but label the investigator as well (Montero, 1977; Warren, 1977). Furthermore, minority researchers may experience difficulties as well as nonminority researchers. Maykovich (1977) has suggested that minority researchers, although appearing to have fewer initial problems, may encounter increased difficulty further into a study.

Problems in Gaining Access

In attempting to gain access to a minority community, the researcher may encounter many barriers (Kahana & Felton, 1977). One barrier is the acceptance and support of the community under study (Kahana & Felton, 1977; Maykovich, 1977; Trimble, 1977; Tsukashima, 1977; Warren, 1977; Weiss, 1977). Failure to secure the cooperation and support of the community under study may result in the community's refusal to participate (Bengston, Grigsby, Corry, & Hruby, 1977). Gaining access to a community is not a one-time occurrence (Warren, 1977); it is a process that entails gaining access to layers of community, friendship circles, social organizations, and underground networks (Adelman, 1986; Warren, 1977).

Survey Methodology and Field Methods: Issues of Design

Numerous methodologists have argued for the use of qualitative methodologies in the study of racial and cultural minorities (Maykovich, 1977; Tsukashima, 1977; Warren, 1977; Weiss, 1977; Zinn, 1979). Although field research was once commonly used in conducting research on ethnic/racial minorities, the development and popularity of survey methodology reshaped the manner in which studies of ethnic/racial minority communities were conducted. Montero (1977) stated that the use of field research techniques "serves to sensitize the investigator to the parameters and nature of the community and its members, including language, customs, and habits that make for a better understanding of a community" (p. 7). Furthermore, field research methodologies suggest an interest in acquiring an in-depth understanding of the structural and cultural organization of an ethnic/racial minority community (Mindel & Kail, 1989). For those studies whose terminal goal is a survey research project, Tsukashima (1977) suggested that the data collected through the use of field research methods can generate questions that later can be tested empirically.

Issues of Measurement

The use of standardized test instruments to collect data on ethnic/racial minority communities may result in problems of reliability and validity. Tests that have been developed and normed on primarily white male samples may not maintain the same levels of reliability and validity when applied to ethnic or racial minority populations (Mindel & Kail, 1989). Biases in the language of a standardized test instrument may detract from the ability to gain a clear understanding of the issues under examination (Tsukashima, 1977) and words may have different meanings for a minority sample or females (Mindel & Kail, 1989). Han (1988), in a study of elderly Korean immigrants, reported that subjects' literal interpretation of a series of given quotes produced significantly different results than a sample of Americans.

A secondary concern worthy of consideration is the gender and ethnicity or race of the researcher. The impact of the insider or outsider issue has been thoroughly discussed throughout the literature (Maykovich, 1977; Merton, 1972; Myers, 1977; Pe-Pua, 1989; Rose, 1978). The use of interviewers who are of divergent ethnic/racial backgrounds from the population under study also may lead to the reliability and validity of the study being questioned (Mindel & Kail, 1989; Myers, 1977; Zinn, 1979).

DIRECTIONS FOR FUTURE RESEARCH

The methodological issues discussed above suggest several implications for the conduct of future research on older lesbians. The following suggestions for increasing the methodological soundness of research on this population are presented as they refer to various stages of the research process: conceptualization, gaining access, and research design.

Conceptualization

Conceptualization has been defined as "the mental process whereby fuzzy and imprecise notions (concepts) are made specific and precise" (Babbie, 1986, p. 554). It is a process through which nominal definitions are assigned to concepts. Operational definitions are developed that will clarify how the concept is to be measured in the real world. Within this process, the theoretical framework and subsequent hypotheses or research questions are developed. It is the theoretical framework that guides the research.

Montero (1977) cautioned that "particular sensitivity to formulating relevant theoretical propositions regarding minority populations" should be used (p. 7). In the study of older women, Calasanti (1992) stated that researchers must explore the "intersection of gender and age" (p. 280). In the study of older lesbians, however, the formulation of theoretical propositions must not only explore the intersection of gender and age, but of homosexuality as well.

Within traditional gerontological literature, gender is treated as a variable and ignores the "structural processes that shape the lived experiences of people" (Calasanti, 1992, p. 280). Recently, however, some gerontologists have attempted to gain an understanding of women's experience of aging by attempting to see gender as a part of a social structure and not just a variable (Allen & Chin-Sang, 1991; Boyd & Tedrick, 1992). Feminists, however, have been insensitive to age as a structural process (Calasanti, 1992; Copper, 1988; MacDonald & Rich, 1983), "nor has the lesbian feminist movement that has supplied the energy and analysis for breaking down so many false barriers between women . . . yet begun to chip away at the wall separating young women from old" (MacDonald & Rich, 1983, p. 46).

If merging the theoretical underpinnings of aging and gender appears complex (Levy, 1988), then the addition of sexuality as a component merely increases the complexity. However, to break down the barriers between young and old, heterosexual and homosexual, male and female, the labor must begin. To accomplish this task Calasanti (1992) has argued for the adoption of a socialist-feminist perspective that captures the diversity and subjectivity of the experiences of women.

Sampling and Gaining Access

Ideally, among a "visible" population, the goal of sampling should result in a pool of participants that represents the population (Babbie, 1986). However, older lesbians are far from being a "visible" population. Kehoe (1986) has referred to this group of women as a "triply invisible minority," referring to the characteristics of age, gender, and sexuality (p. 139). The issue, then, remains how to gain access to the estimated 1,100,880 lesbians in the United States who are older than 65 years.

Over the past several years, numerous organizations have formed to meet the needs of older lesbians, including Older Women's League, Lavender Panthers, The Society of Gay and Lesbian Senior Citizens, Slightly Older Lesbians, Gays Over 40, and Senior Action in a Gay Environment. The gaining of support and cooperation from these organizations and other lesbian support networks can facilitate entry into the "secret world" of the older lesbian. However, women who choose to avail themselves of the services offered by these organizations have, for the most part, been able to break the walls of oppression and stigmatization of labels. These are the women who are most easily identified in the studies of older lesbians. Few studies, however, have been able to open the lace curtains to those women who do not identify themselves as lesbians. Researchers who have been able to break the barriers have done so by earning the trust and support of numerous layers of social networks (Warren, 1977). Unfortunately, those researchers who have parted the lace curtains, have reported on predominately white older women.

The question remains: How does a researcher find the path to lesbians of color? Lesbian organizations exist that are designed to meet the age-specific needs of older lesbians as do groups whose purpose is to meet the needs of lesbians of color. As with their white peers, the women who participate in these organizations have, for the most part, overcome oppression. The disadvantage to this route may be the low number of older women who participate. However, contacts in the social networks and friendship circles of other women of color can lead to the identification of older lesbians of color.

Research Design

This phase of research entails development of a plan through which the study will be implemented. Much of the published research on older lesbians has focused on literature reviews and the development of conceptual frameworks and theoretical orientations. Research that has involved use of a methodological application has been evenly split, with the focus on use of survey methodology (Kehoe, 1986, 1988; and Lucco, 1987) and structured interviews (Berger, 1984; Minnigerode & Adelman, 1978; Tully, 1989). Other methodologies that have been used have included content analysis (Riege-Laner, 1979) and life review (Galassi, 1991).

The need for innovative methods of sample collection exists as does the need for innovative methods for data collection. Copper (1988) and MacDonald and Rich (1983), in their discussion of ageism within the lesbian community, identified lesbians' need to be heard and respected and their need to communicate with women with whom they could "be comfortably intimate–women [they] can trust" (Copper, 1988, p. 33). What has been identified is a need for a methodology that not only will allow the researchers to have their questions answered but will enable the older lesbians who partici-pate in the study to feel as if they have had an opportunity to discuss what is also important to them, and also to experience a sense of communal support.

Maykovich (1977) has suggested that the use of qualitative meth-odologies can identify theoretical clues that later can be tested em-pirically. Furthermore, Pe-Pua (1989) has discussed the use of a Filipino methodology, *Pagatanong-tanong,* which has been used in cross-cultural studies. Pagatanong-tanong has four basic character-istics, which appear to meet the expressed needs of Copper (1988) and MacDonald and Rich (1983):

> (1) It is participatory in nature; the informant has input in the structure of the interaction in terms of defining its direction and time management; (2) The researcher and the informant are equal in status; both parties may ask each other questions for about the same length of time; (3) It is appropriate and adaptive to the conditions of the group of informants in that it conforms to existing group norms; and (4) It is integrated with other indigenous research methods. (Pe-Pua, 1989, p. 147)

It is through such innovative methodologies that perhaps re-searchers can find that middle ground where older lesbians feel as if they have an opportunity to share their wisdom and researchers are able to receive and understand that wisdom. Many of the issues illustrated throughout this article may not appear to be specific to older lesbians. However, the historical and social influences of their past continue to affect who they are, how they define themselves, and to what extent they hide their relationships. Perhaps, in time, researchers will be able to find ways to resolve these and other issues.

REFERENCES

Adelman, M. (1986). *Long time passing: Lives of older lesbians.* Boston: Alyson.

Adelman, M. (1990). Stigma, gay lifestyles, and adjustment to aging: A study of later-life gay men and lesbians. *Journal of Homosexuality, 20*(3/4), 7-32.

Allen, K. R., & Chin-Sang, V. (1991). A lifetime of work: The context and meanings of leisure for aging black women. *Gerontologist, 30*(6), 734-740.

Babbie, E. (1986). *The practice of social research* (4th ed.). Belmont, CA: Wadsworth.

Barrett, M. B. (1989). *Invisible lives: The truth about millions of women-loving women.* New York: William Morrow.

Bell, A. P. (1975). Research in homosexuality: Back to the drawing board. *Archives of Sexual Behavior, 4*(4), 421-431.

Bengston, V. L., Grigsby, E., Corry, E. M., & Hruby, M. (1977). Relating academic research to community concerns: A case study in collaborative effort. *Journal of Social Issues, 33*(4), 75-92.

Berger, R. M. (1982). The unseen minority: Older gays and lesbians. *Social Work, 27,* 236-242.

Berger, R. M. (1984). Realities of gay and lesbian aging. *Social Work, 29,* 57-62.

Boyd, R., & Tedrick, T. (1992, October). *Leisure in the lives of older black women.* Paper presented at the meeting of the National Recreation and Parks Association, Leisure Research Symposium, Cincinnati, OH.

Calasanti, T. M. (1992). Theorizing about gender and aging: Beginning with the voices of women. *Gerontologist, 32*(2), 280-282.

Chafetz, J. S., Sampson, P., Beck, P., & West, J. (1974). A study of homosexual women. *Social Work, 19,* 714-723.

Copper, B. (1988). *Over the hill: Reflections on ageism between women.* Freedom, CA: The Crossing Press.

Cruikshank, M. (1990). Lavender and gray: A brief survey of lesbian and gay aging studies. *Journal of Homosexuality, 20*(3/4), 77-88.

Galassi, F. S. (1991). A life review workshop for gay and lesbian elders. *Journal of Gerontological Social Work, 16*(1/2), 75-86.

Han, S. (1988). The relationship between life satisfaction and flow in elderly Korean immigrants. In M. Csikszentmihalyi & I. S. Csikszentmihalyi (Eds.), *Optimal experience: Psychological studies of flow consciousness* (pp. 138-149). New York: Cambridge University Press.

Harry, J. (1986). Sampling gay men. *Journal of Sex Research, 22*(1), 21-34.

Henderson, K. A., Bialeschki, M. D., Shaw, S., & Freysinger, V. (1989). *A leisure of one's own: A feminist perspective on women's leisure.* State College, PA: Venture Publishing.

Kahana, E., & Felton, B. J. (1977). Social context and personal need: A study of Polish and Jewish aged. *Journal of Social Issues, 33*(4), 56-74.

Kehoe, M. (1986). Lesbians over 65: A triply invisible minority. *Journal of Homosexuality, 12*(3/4), 139-152.

Kehoe, M. (1988). Lesbians over 60 speak for themselves. *Journal of Homosexuality, 16*(3/4), 1-111.

Kinsey, A. C., Pomeroy, W. B., Martin, C. R., & Gebhard, P. H. (1953). *Sexual behavior in the human female.* Philadelphia: W. B. Saunders.

Levy, J. A. (1988). Intersections of gender and aging. *Sociological Quarterly, 29*, 479-486.

Leznoff, M. (1956). Interviewing homosexuals. *Archives of Sexual Behavior, 62*(2), 202-204.

Lucco, A. J. (1987). Planned retirement housing preferences of older homosexuals. *Journal of Homosexuality, 14*(3/4), 35-56.

MacDonald, B., & Rich, C. (1983). *Look me in the eye. Old women, aging, and ageism.* San Francisco: Spinsters Ink.

Martin, D., & Lyon, P. (1972). *Lesbian/woman.* New York: Bantam.

Maykovich, M. K. (1977). The difficulties of a minority researcher in minority communities. *Journal of Social Issues, 33*(4), 108-119.

Merton, R. K. (1972). Insiders and outsiders: A chapter in the sociology of knowledge. *American Journal of Sociology, 78*, 9-47.

Mindel, C. H., & Kail, B. L. (1989). Issues in research on the older woman of color. *Journal of Drug Issues, 19*(2), 191-206.

Minnigerode, F. A., & Adelman, M. R. (1978). Elderly homosexual women and men: Report on a pilot study. *Family Coordinator, 27*(4), 451-456.

Montero, D. (1977). Research among racial and cultural minorities: An overview. *Journal of Social Issues, 3*(4), 1-10.

Morales, E. S. (1990). Ethnic minority families and minority gays and lesbians. *Marriage and Family Review, 14*(3/4), 217-239.

Myers, V. (1977). Survey methods for minority populations. *Journal of Social Issues, 33*(4), 11-19.

Pe-Pua, R. (1989). Pagatanong-tanong: A cross-cultural research method. *International Journal of Intercultural Relations, 13*(2), 147-163.

Poor, M. (1982). The older lesbian. In M. Cruikshank (Ed.), *Lesbian studies* (pp. 165-173). Old Westbury, NY: Feminist Press.

Raphael, S., & Robinson, M. (1984). The older lesbian: Love relationships and friendship patterns. In T. Darty & S. Potter (Eds.), *Women-identified women* (pp. 67-82). Palo Alto, CA: Mayfield.

Riege-Laner, M. (1979). Growing older female: Heterosexual and homosexual. *Journal of Homosexuality, 4*(3), 267-275.

Rose, P. I. (1978). *"Nobody knows the trouble I've seen": Some reflections on the insider outsider debate.* Northampton, MA: Smith College.

Trimble, J. E. (1977). The sojourner in the American Indian community: Methodological issues and concerns. *Journal of Social Issues, 33*(4), 159-174.

Tsukashima, R. T. (1977). Merging fieldwork and survey research in the study of a minority community. *Journal of Social Issues, 33*(4), 133-143.

Tully, C. T. (1989). Caregiving: What do midlife lesbians view as important? *Journal of Gay & Lesbian Psychotherapy, 1*(1), 87-103.

U. S. Department of Commerce, Bureau of the Census. (1991). *Statistical abstracts of the United States: 1991* (111th ed.). Washington, DC: U.S. Government Printing Office.

Warren, C. A. (1977). Fieldwork in the gay world: Issues in phenomenological research. *Journal of Social Issues, 33*(4), 93-107.

Weinberg, M. (1970). Homosexual samples: Differences and similarities. *Journal of Sex Research, 6*(4), 312-325.

Weiss, C. H. (1977). Survey researchers and minority communities. *Journal of Social Issues, 33*(4), 20-35.

Wolf, D. C. (1978, November). Close friendship patterns of older lesbians. Paper presented at the annual convention of the Gerontological Society of America, Dallas, TX.

Zinn, M. B. (1979). Field research in minority communities: Ethical, methodological, and political observations by an insider. *Social Problems, 27*(2), 209-219.

Research in Lesbian Communities:
Ethical Dilemmas

Natalie Jane Woodman
Carol T. Tully
Chrystal C. Barranti

SUMMARY. In this paper the authors address the three major areas in which ethical dilemmas may be experienced by those who do research in lesbian communities: (1) confidentiality, (2) anonymity, and (3) professional boundaries. Lesbian researchers who use the most common method of gathering data on lesbians–the snowball sampling technique–may encounter ethical dilemmas when conducting research in lesbian communities. In addition, the authors identify related questions that lesbian investigators must consider. Possible solutions to these dilemmas include expanding the sampling frame, using more explicit consent forms, and honoring the power and privilege inherent in the professional role as researcher.

Newspapers publish the names of those who have violated professional ethical standards (National Association of Social Workers [NASW], 1993); schools of social work are mandated to include

Natalie Jane Woodman, MSS, ACSW, ICSW, is Professor Emerita at the School of Social Work, Arizona State University, 6722 North 23rd Place, Phoenix, AZ 85106. Carol T. Tully, PhD, is Associate Professor at Tulane School of Social Work, Tulane University, New Orleans, LA 70118-5672. Chrystal C. Barranti, PhD, is Therapy Services Coordinator at the Center for Mental Health, West Paces Medical Center, Atlanta, GA 30327.

[Haworth co-indexing entry note]: "Research in Lesbian Communities: Ethical Dilemmas." Woodman, Natalie Jane, Carol T. Tully, and Chrystal C. Barranti. Co-published simultaneously in *Journal of Gay & Lesbian Social Services* (The Haworth Press, Inc.) Vol. 3, No. 1, 1995, pp. 57-66; and: *Lesbian Social Services: Research Issues* (ed: Carol T. Tully) The Haworth Press, Inc., 1995, pp. 57-66; and: *Lesbian Social Services: Research Issues* (ed: Carol T. Tully) Harrington Park Press, an imprint of The Haworth Press, Inc., 1995, pp. 57-66. Multiple copies of this article/chapter may be purchased from The Haworth Document Delivery Center [1-800-3-HAWORTH; 9:00 a.m. - 5:00 p.m. (EST)].

57

professional values and ethics as part of their accreditation standards (Council on Social Work Education [CSWE], 1992); human subject review panels stress the importance of ethical research (Institutional Review Board, 1991); research texts include content related to ethics (Bailey, 1987; Corcoran & Fischer, 1987; Gibbs, 1991; Rubin & Babbie, 1993); and even texts associated with statistical software packages include information related to the ethics of research (Norusis, 1988). Yet, although there seem to be appropriate standards regarding the ethical deportment of professionals (Bailey, 1987; NASW, 1979; Rubin & Babbie, 1993), the literature is filled with examples of ethical misconduct (Henig, 1992; Landers, 1992) and discussions of ethical dilemmas (Edelwich & Brodsky, 1982; Peterson, 1992).

With the continuing focus on appropriate ethical behavior in practice and research, one area that has never been specifically examined in the literature is that of ethical dilemmas encountered by lesbians who conduct research with other lesbians in their community. Using what has become the most common sampling method to collect data across all age groups–the non-probability snowball or chain referral sampling method (Albro & Tully, 1977; Dancey, 1992; Kehoe, 1988; Schneider, 1989; Tully, 1989; Woodman, 1992; Woodman & Lenna, 1980), lesbian researchers who conduct research using lesbian samples may face ethical dilemmas in the areas of confidentiality, protection of respondents' anonymity, and professional boundaries. In this article, the authors identify these major obstacles to research, discuss related questions that researchers must consider, and suggest solutions.

ETHICAL DILEMMAS

Confidentiality

Protection of participant confidentiality is one of the ethical hallmarks in conducting research with any population. For example, the NASW (1979) *Code of Ethics* clearly delineates that "the social worker should respect the privacy of clients and hold in confidence all information obtained in the course of professional service"

(p. 2). In addition, human subject review boards require anonymity or confidentiality to protect all research subjects (Institutional Review Board, 1991). How, then, does the area of confidentiality pose particular ethical dilemmas for lesbian researchers who conduct research in lesbian communities? Perhaps one of the predominant factors affecting the probability of ethical dilemmas is the smallness of the lesbian community and the almost unavoidable overlapping of roles by researchers and participants alike. This reality poses several questions related to research participants and to the quality of the research data. For example, in using the often narrowly defined lesbian community as a research focus, to what extent do research subjects feel secure in the assurance of confidentiality when, subsequent to the data gathering, they expect to encounter the researcher in social settings?

Since the 1970s, research has revealed that subjects who participate in research studies conducted within the lesbian community often provide unsolicited information related to the research project when the researcher encounters them in social settings following the initial data gathering process (Woodman, 1992; Woodman & Lenna, 1980). Subjects have reported that they give additional information related to the specific focus of the research in nonstructured and non-research settings because they feel more relaxed and have come to trust the researcher more in a social setting than in a structured interview (Woodman, 1992; Woodman & Lenna, 1980). This phenomenon does not seem time related–subjects have presented additional data related to a specific study, days, weeks, or months following the initial research data gathering phase (Woodman, 1992; Woodman & Lenna, 1980).

Given this reality, to what extent can researchers in the lesbian community who happen to be members of that community have confidence in the validity and reliability of the data that are originally gathered? Although being a member of a community under study may help establish face validity (Bailey, 1987; Rubin & Babbie, 1993), the need to test for external validity is important. Testing for external validity remains a more formidable task; however, establishing reliability may be somewhat less problematic, especially if data generated from one study are consistent with other similar samples. For example, inasmuch as studies of lesbian samples continue to generate similar data, the measurement instruments and data seem to be at least reliable, if not externally valid (Lott-White-head, 1992).

Although some (Rogers & Shoemaker, 1971) may argue that the best communication and hence the best data gathering occurs between persons who are alike, this concept of homophily presents a dilemma for lesbian researchers who conduct research in their own communities. How does the researcher block out content obtained in a research setting from information received in a social sphere? How does the researcher instill confidence in the research subject that confidentiality is guaranteed when there is overlapping of roles and a smallness of community? Simply, it is vital that lesbian researchers who study those with whom they socially interact must maintain a constant vigil not to divulge findings obtained in a research setting beyond that context. The research process and data must be as confidential to the researcher as is the therapeutic relationship between the client and the therapist. However tempting it may be to carry the role and status of researcher into the social setting, unless the study involves ethnography, the researcher who does cross this boundary and blurs role contexts is in violation of professional ethical standards that govern the research process (Gillespie, 1987).

Anonymity

The concept of confidentiality between the researcher and study participants is merely one issue associated with the protection of the sample. *Anonymity,* that is, keeping the identities of the sample unknown, also becomes an issue when using a snowball or chain referral sampling process. Practicing anonymity can be considered a challenge when the conditions of a small oppressed community and multiple overlapping roles–all typical characteristics of the lesbian researcher-lesbian community experience–are present. In such instances, the ability to protect anonymity can be a considerable challenge. For instance, it is common for lesbians who participate as research subjects, to express an eagerness to read the study's results (Woodman, 1992). Although the subject's right to have access to the final draft of the study is a standard in research practice, a particular dilemma arises in relation to the protection of anonymity. For example, given the smallness and the closeness of the lesbian community, even with the careful elimination of names in the write-up, it may be possible to identify participants through demographic data published in the results. In addition to interest in identifying participants, the desire to read final results has been motivated by a wish to know what others in the community have said (Woodman, 1992). Although this curiosity may reflect a healthy desire for the affirmation that comes from the simple fact that a research study acknowledges the existence of the lesbian community and lesbian identity, the issue of how to protect anonymity remains.

Explanations of professional responsibility during the research process require considerable reinforcement. Although promises of anonymity or confidentiality are made in good faith, it is essential that researchers use formal processes such as code numbers in lieu of participant names. Subjects' identities should not in any way be shared beyond the research boundaries. Given the defining characteristics of the lesbian community, research with this population may require researchers to become even more creative when disguising respondent identity, without contaminating the data.

It is important that researchers have some control over protecting participants' anonymity; however, researchers have little control over participants themselves. For instance, in one research project within a lesbian community, all the research subjects celebrated their contributions to the research project by having a dinner together (Woodman, 1992). In another instance, research participants were all part of a women's dance that was held during the research process (Woodman, 1992). Although researchers specify the issues of anonymity and confidentiality with research participants during the research project, perhaps researchers in the lesbian community need to broaden the parameters of these ethical considerations to the entire community in which they are conducting their study.

Professional Boundaries

Theoretically, researchers embark on studies with an objective neutrality that is fueled by scholarly inquiry and guided by ethical principles. Whereas in principle, the role of the researcher is well defined, that role can become blurred when placed within the context of a small and close community in which multiple roles often overlap. The lesbian researcher conducting research in her own lesbian community may also be the study participant's therapist, professor, friend, co-worker, or teammate. However, it is this reality of multiple and overlapping roles that may give the lesbian researcher both advantage and challenge. As a member of the lesbian community, the researcher may have a point of entry that is inaccessible to non-lesbians. Participants may more easily trust and give responses to interviews or questionnaires that they would not otherwise give to "outsiders." In addition, as a member of the minority culture which she is researching, the lesbian investigator may have a keener sense of the significant questions needing exploration. She may also have a more meaningful and appropriate context out of which to interpret results—one that is unavailable to the heterosexual researcher.

Although the existence of multiple overlapping roles has its advantages, it is imperative that investigators assume responsibility for acknowledging and protecting the professional boundaries inherent in the privileged role of researcher. The existence of these multiple overlapping roles makes the vigilance of professional boundaries especially significant. For example, if the investigator learns through the interview process that a research participant is single and enjoys hobbies similar to the researcher's single friend, does the investigator share this information with her friend who is seeking a relationship? Does the investigator who is also a therapist use her power to solicit participants from her clinical practice? Does a researcher express her academic prowess in a social setting by divulging confidential information gained in her research process? Given the mandate to protect and to enhance the dignity and well-being of each individual served (National Federation of Societies for Clinical Social Work, 1988), the response to these boundary dilemmas must be an emphatic "no!"

With professional position comes power and privilege. Acknowledging this power and privilege is a must if researchers are to protect professional boundaries and conduct ethical research practice in the lesbian community. Without the acknowledgement and acceptance of the responsibility of professional power and privilege, the probability for unethical practice is present (Peterson, 1992). Perhaps at the heart of all ethical dilemmas faced by lesbian researchers who do research in their lesbian communities is this concept of maintaining professional boundaries in the midst of a small minority community in which multiple overlapping roles are the norm. When researchers are able to maintain professional boundaries with integrity, they may more confidently protect confidentiality and anonymity within ethical guidelines.

POSSIBLE SOLUTIONS

Confidentiality, anonymity, and professional boundaries are directly related to the greater research dilemma of researcher membership in the community being studied. Although these areas may pose little problem for ethical dilemmas in ethnography or ethnomethodological studies, they warrant significant attention for survey research methods and quasi-experimental or experimental research designs. Three solutions to overcoming the ethical dilemmas present in these areas are readily apparent.

First, lesbians could abandon the role of researcher within their lesbian culture and leave the task to heterosexuals or gay men. Second, lesbian researchers could confine their research to lesbian communities far removed from their own communities. Third, researchers could make lesbian research subjects more aware of these ethical issues through appropriate informed consent before their participation in the research.

A paucity of information related to lesbian issues continues to exist, and those studies that have examined the lesbian community have been conducted primarily by lesbians themselves (Tully, 1983). Nevertheless, can minority group members obtain reliable information from their own communities? Within the social work community exists a group that advocates that valid research of minority groups can and ought to be conducted with only minority group members. For example, Smith (1973) has argued that valid minority research can only be accomplished by a minority group member because group membership is necessary to assure that no cultural biases exist within the researcher that would distort the findings. Furthermore, minority status is essential if the researcher is to gain access and acceptance by a minority community.

Tully (1994) has pointed out that because the lesbian community is largely invisible within the heterosexual culture, researchers outside the community will naively overlook the majority of the lesbian community by seeing only what the lesbian community chooses to share with the majority culture. Additionally, because homophobia plays such a significant role in the lives of lesbians (Herek, 1990), it is difficult for heterosexuals (even women) to gain access to the lesbian community for research purposes (Lott-Whitehead, 1992). Thus, the development of appropriate research questions, adequate sampling, and valid findings become difficult if not impossible for non-lesbians.

Assuming that valid research within the lesbian community can be conducted by lesbians who are part of that community, how is this best accomplished? There seem to be two probable solutions that allow for ethical research. Lesbian researchers who use survey research methods can expand their sampling frame to include those outside their personal communities. This deliberate expansion of the sampling frame ensures a more diverse sample and, coupled with explicit informed consent forms, can alleviate the aforementioned ethical dilemmas. Those wishing to conduct quasi-experimental or experimental studies closer to home can also avoid or at least identify for participants ethical dilemmas by using explicit informed consent forms that simply detail the roles of the researcher and the participant, as well as the rules for the study.

In conducting any research within the lesbian community, lesbian researchers must develop an explicit informed consent. This becomes fairly easy in the case of mailed questionnaires because respondents' anonymity can be assured, especially if they come from a widely diverse geographic area. When the research participants' identities are made known to researchers, it is imperative that researchers inform participants that, although the data will be confidential, there may be some instances in which confidentiality cannot be absolutely assured. For example, in the case of research within small lesbian communities, researchers must inform participants that the researchers will keep the data confidential; however, respondents, too, have an obligation to keep their responses private and unique situations or characteristics of a respondent or her situation that are generally known in the lesbian community may render confidentiality moot.

Finally, it is critical that lesbian researchers acknowledge and honor both the power and privilege inherent in the professional role as researcher. Even amidst multiple overlapping roles, researchers must maintain the professional boundary of the researcher/participant by scrupulously protecting confidentiality and anonymity. Further honoring of the boundary might include refraining from discussing the research project or its findings in social settings until the study is published or the researcher has held a debriefing meeting in the community. Significantly, researchers can assure the honoring of the boundary by not using data and information gained through the research project for personal gain in any way.

It is imperative that realistic knowledge of the lesbian community be generated through the continuation of empirically based research. The most appropriate persons to conduct such research seem to be lesbian researchers who are aware of the pitfalls of their endeavors, and who have brought into full consciousness the responsibility to adhere to ethical principles for social science research.

REFERENCES

Albro, J. C., & Tully, C. T. (1977). A study of lesbian lifestyles in the homosexual micro-culture and the heterosexual macro-culture. *Journal of Homosexuality,* *4*(4), 331-344.

Bailey, K. D. (1987). *Methods of social research* (3rd ed.). New York: The Free Press.

Corcoran, K., & Fischer, J. (1987). *Measures for clinical practice: A sourcebook.* New York: The Free Press.

Council on Social Work Education. (1992). *Handbook of accreditation standards and procedures.* Alexandria, VA: Author.

Dancey, C. P. (1992). The relationship of instrumentality and expressivity. *Journal of Homosexuality, 23*(4), 71-82.

Edelwich, J., & Brodsky, A. (1982). *Sexual dilemmas for the helping professional.* New York: Brunner/Mazel.

Gibbs, L. E. (1991). *Scientific reasoning for social workers: Bridging the gap between research and practice.* New York: Merrill.

Gillespie, D. F. (1987). Ethical issues in research. In A. Minihan (Ed.), *Encyclopedia of social work* (18th Ed., pp. 503-512). Silver Spring, MD: National Association of Social Workers.

Henig, R. M. (1992, November). Ethicists mull challenges to societal values. *AARP Bulletin,* pp. 2, 13.

Herek, G. (1990). Homophobia. In W. B. Dynes (Ed.), *Encyclopedia of homosexuality* (pp. 552-555). New York: Garland Publishing.

Institutional Review Board. (1991). *Instructions for investigators conducting research with human participants.* Athens: The University of Georgia.

Kehoe, M. (1988). Lesbians over 60 speak for themselves. *Journal of Homosexuality, 16*(3/4), 1-111.

Landers, S. (1992, October). Ethical boundaries easily trespassed. *NASW News,* p. 3.

Lott-Whitehead, L. (1992). *The families of lesbian mothers.* Master's Thesis, The University of Georgia, Athens.

National Association of Social Workers. (1979). *Code of ethics.* Silver Spring, MD: Author.

National Association of Social Workers. (1993, July). Sanctions in force. *NASW News,* p. 8.

National Federation of Societies for Clinical Social Work. (1988). *Code of ethics.* Arlington, VA: Author.

Norusis, M. J. (1988). *SPSS/PC+ Studentwear.* Chicago: SPSS.

Peterson, M. R. (1992). *At personal risk: Boundary violations in professional-client relationships.* New York: W. W. Norton.

Rogers, E. M., & Shoemaker, F. F. (1971). *Communication of innovations: A cross-cultural approach.* New York: Free Press.

Rubin, A., & Babbie, E. (1993). *Research methods for social work* (2nd Ed.). Pacific Grove, CA: Brooks/Cole.

Schneider, M. (1989). Sappho was a right-on adolescent: Growing up lesbian. *Journal of Homosexuality, 17*(1/2), 111-130.

Smith, N. F. (1973). Who should do minority research? *Social Casework, 54*(7), 393-397.

Tully, C. T. (1989). Caregiving: What do midlife lesbians view as important? *Journal of Gay & Lesbian Psychotherapy, 1*(1), 87-103.

Tully, C. T. (1994). Should only gay and lesbian organizers operate in the lesbian and gay community? In M. J. Austin and J. I. Lowe (Eds.), *Controversial issues in communities and organizations: Perspectives on macro-practice* (pp. 86-96). Boston: Allyn and Bacon.

Tully, C. T. (1983). *Social support systems of a selected sample of older women.* Unpublished doctoral dissertation, Virginia Commonwealth University, Richmond, VA.

Woodman, N. J., & Lenna, H. R. (1980). *Counseling with gay men and women.* San Francisco: Jossey-Bass.

Woodman, N. J. (1992). Personal research notes. Unpublished.

Fusion and Conflict Resolution in Lesbian Relationships

Vickie Causby
Lettie Lockhart
Barbara White
Kathryn Greene

SUMMARY. In this study the authors explore the issues of social distancing and conflict resolution in lesbian relationships. The authors surveyed 275 lesbians about the extent of fusion in their relationships, sources of conflict, and styles of conflict resolution. Results with a nonclinical sample indicated that lesbians reported moderate levels of fusion in their relationships. Furthermore, two subscales of fusion–fusion time issues and sharing–were produced from these data. Sharing large amounts of time with lesbian partners apparently was not problematic for many couples. However, sharing concrete items (e.g., money, clothing, or car) and professional services (e.g., physician or therapist) made maintaining appropriate boundaries more difficult. Participants who reported high sharing fusion tended to report more sources of conflict and poorer conflict resolution strategies with their partners, including physical aggression and violence.

Vickie Causby, PhD, is Associate Professor at the School of Social Work, East Carolina University, Greenville, NC 27858-4353. Lettie Lockhart, PhD, is Associate Professor at the School of Social Work, University of Georgia, Athens, GA 30602-7016. Barbara White, PhD, is Professor at the School of Social Work, University of Texas at Austin, Austin, TX 78712-1703. Kathryn Greene, PhD, is Assistant Professor in the Department of Communications, East Carolina University, Greenville, NC 27858-4353.

[Haworth co-indexing entry note]: "Fusion and Conflict Resolution in Lesbian Relationships." Causby, Vickie et al. Co-published simultaneously in *Journal of Gay & Lesbian Social Services* (The Haworth Press, Inc.) Vol. 3, No. 1, 1995, pp. 67-82; and: *Lesbian Social Services: Research Issues* (ed: Carol T. Tully) The Haworth Press, Inc., 1995, pp. 67-82; and: *Lesbian Social Services: Research Issues* (ed: Carol T. Tully) Harrington Park Press, an imprint of The Haworth Press, Inc., 1995, pp. 67-82. Multiple copies of this article/chapter may be purchased from The Haworth Document Delivery Center [1-800-3-HAWORTH; 9:00 a.m. - 5:00 p.m. (EST)].

For well over a decade, lesbian couples have been described as fused, enmeshed, or merged (Douglas, 1990; Krestan & Bepko, 1980; Pearlman, 1989; Peplau, Cochran, Rook, & Padesky, 1978; Zacks, Green, & Marrow, 1988). The assumption is that fusion, merger, or enmeshment creates dysfunctional relationships through poor conflict resolution, conflicts over time spent with anyone outside the relationship, low self-esteem, and isolation. The first set of obstacles for young lesbians, according to Berg-Cross (1988), involves the dual developmental tasks of "coming out" and escaping the suffocating fusion typical of many lesbian relationships. Lesbians are seen as cutting themselves off from others in a two-against-the-world posture (Caldwell & Peplau, 1984; Krestan & Bepko, 1980; Pearlman, 1989).

The level of fusion in all lesbian relationships is assumed to be extremely high and therefore dysfunctional. Both assumptions–that fusion in lesbian relationships is high and that high levels of fusion are dysfunctional–may be unfounded. Numerous authors have cited extreme levels of fusion in lesbian couples and have defined the level of dependence as a problem, even though the couples also reported high levels of satisfaction with their relationships (Eldridge & Gilbert, 1990; Kurdek, 1992; Peplau, Padesky, & Hamilton, 1983). In a nonclinical population, can fusion be seen as an adaptable strength rather than a pathological symptom for lesbian couples?

This article presents a literature review that defines fusion and provides an overview of the extent of fusion reported in lesbian relationships. Previously cited theoretical reasons for greater fusion or enmeshment with lesbians are discussed. This article also addresses conflict styles, sources of conflict, and means of conflict resolution. Finally, the authors present the findings of a study on fusion in lesbian relationships.

LITERATURE REVIEW

Fusion, Enmeshment, and Merger

Peplau and her colleagues (1978) have pointed out that in all close relationships, a balancing of the desire for intimacy and the desire for independence is required. The effort to achieve a satisfactory pattern of separateness and connectedness is a fundamental, lifelong task for couples, regardless of sexual orientation. Fusion, enmeshment, and merger are terms that have been used to describe the emotional relationship between lesbian couples. These terms have been used interchangeably to identify a psychological state in which there is a loss of oneself as an individual and also a state of imbeddedness in, or undifferentiation within, the relational context (Berg-Cross, 1988; Krestan & Bepko, 1980; Pearlman, 1989). Merged partners find it difficult or even undesirable to think, act, or feel separately from each other (Burch, 1982).

The concept of boundaries is essential in understanding the nature of fusion. Minuchin (1974) defined *boundaries* of a subsystem as the rules used to define who participates in the subsystem and how they participate. This task of defining the inner and outer boundaries of a couple involves deciding how emotionally close one partner can come before there is a loss of individuality. The function of boundaries is to protect the differentiation of the system. The boundaries of a couple must be clear enough to allow individuals to carry out their functions without undue interference, but those boundaries must also allow contrast between both members of the couple (Minuchin, 1974).

Reasons for High Levels of Fusion in Lesbian Relationships

Many theories have explained why high levels of fusion continue to be cited in lesbian relationships. From a systems perspective, it has been hypothesized that couples fuse as a response to a hostile environment (Krestan & Bepko, 1980). Lesbian couples turn to each other for validation and support of the relationship that they do not often get from the larger society. Consequently, they may have relatively closed boundaries. Unlike lesbian or gay couples, heterosexual couples receive feedback regarding boundaries and rules that are normative and necessary to individual functioning (Zacks, Green, & Marrow, 1988).

Moreover, families, friends, and co-workers may fail to treat two women as a couple. This lack of affirmation is further exacerbated by the absence of rituals and legal sanctions. Without outside boundaries, the lesbian couple tends to create its own boundaries through intense involvement and exclusion of others (Krestan & Bepko, 1980; Pearlman, 1989).

In contrast to a systems perspective, Pearlman (1989) hypothesized that lesbian couples get stuck in the first stage of couple development, or "limerance" which is characterized by intense bonding, and the loss of ego boundaries and individuality. In the second stage of couple development, the power or control stage, couples struggle with issues of differentiation and dependency. At this point, they begin to reestablish individual boundaries. Lesbian couples who deny differences and avoid conflict tend to return to a more merger-like state (Pearlman, 1989).

Other explanations of why fusion problems are frequently associated with lesbian relationships have related to the psychosocial development of women and to the socialization of lesbians as women. Chodorow's (1978) work has been cited frequently as a comprehensive explanation of gender differences. She stated that the psychological separation of the child from the mother is never as complete for girls as it is for boys. Consequently, ego boundaries are less tightly formed, so women have more difficulty seeing themselves as separate individuals. This psychological differentiation places women at a greater tendency toward fusion or merger in intimate relationships, regardless of their sexual orientation. Furthermore, when the maternal expectation of the daughter is one of sameness with the mother and daughters do not conform (i.e., because of lesbian behavior), mothers react by emotionally distancing the daughter (Pearlman, 1989). Distancing then begins to mean disapproval and is connected with relationship loss. These relationship patterns may shape the dynamics for future relationships with women, especially in lesbian relationships.

Although dependency needs are one of the universal aspects of relationships, there is a widespread inclination to believe that women have greater dependency needs than men. Women are socialized to focus on relationships and to depend on others (Berg-Cross, 1988). Some authors may believe it is women who have low feelings of personal efficacy. For example, Lerner (1989) indicated that women may fear that men or their main relationships will not tolerate increases in autonomous functioning, especially as long as there is the possibility of obtaining dependent, compliant relationships.

Fusion for lesbians, then, may be a response to homophobia from the larger community as well as lack of affirmation for their boundaries as a couple. The psychosocial development and socialization of lesbians as women also may contribute to higher levels of fusion. Based on this information, one research question for the current study was, *What is the extent of fusion in lesbian relationships when using a nonclinical population?*

Sources of Conflict

The behavioral expression of fusion may be manifested in extreme dependency or in extreme distancing. The more unhappy partner may act out her feelings by having an affair or fantasies of an affair, may provoke quarrels, and may fume with unexpressed anger (Burch, 1982). That partner also may act out a desire for increased separateness through over-involvement with work, increased disappointment with the relationship, or lack of sexual interest (Lindenbaum, 1985; Pearlman, 1989).

Almost an infinite number of issues can serve as possible sources of conflict for persons in intimate relationships. Sources of conflict identified in the conflict and family violence literature indicate that couples argue over issues that are both internal and external to the individuals in the relationship. Sources of internal conflict may include issues of emotional and financial dependency. Gelles and Straus (1978) reported that jealousy and the use of alcohol or drugs are also major sources of conflict in families. Sources of external conflict may consist of issues that cause stress in the family (e.g., unemployment, jobs, and finances). Other stressors for couples may relate to relationships outside the boundaries of the primary couple such as relationships with family, friends, and the partner's children.

Hypothesis 1 in this study was that *lesbians who report higher levels of fusion will report more conflict over internal and relational issues and less conflict over external issues.*

Conflict Styles and Conflict Resolution

Conflict is inevitable in individual lives as well as in close relationships (Lloyd, 1990; Roloff, 1987). Interpersonal conflict involves communication about incompatible goals and strategies used to manage differences (Canary, Cunningham, & Cody, 1988). Given that communication is one avenue of conflict resolution, interpersonal communication can function as a means of resource exchange and also as a means for couples to produce relationship rewards (Roloff, 1987).

Conflict styles comprise two partially competing goals: (a) concern for oneself and (b) concern for another person (Hocker & Wilmot, 1985). Sillars' (1980) work used a three-dimensional model to assess individual conflict styles. Those three styles were: (a) passive-indirect (avoidance, accommodation, and nonconfrontation); (b) integrative (managing conflict with a win-win strategy); and (c) distributive (forceful, controlling tactics from a competitive win-lose orientation). Similarly, Covey (1989) perceived that conflict is addressed by six paradigms of human interaction: "win-win," "win-lose," "lose-win," "lose-lose," "win," and "win-win" or "no deal." He stated that the paradigms of human interaction operate on a maturity continuum from dependence to independence to interdependence.

In terms of conflict style and gender, Canary, Cunningham and Cody (1988) indicated that, although research on the use of conflict styles based on gender is inconclusive, women are more likely to select strategies that maintain positive feelings and relationships. Women use styles that are more consistent with problem-solving strategies and are integrative in nature (Greene, Parker, & Serovich, 1992).

Violence as a Means of Conflict Resolution

Like Sillars (1980) and Covey (1989), Straus (1979) examined conflict resolution tactics, specifically what Sillars (1980) labeled as distributive or violence tactics used in families. One tactic, verbal aggression, is the "use of verbal and nonverbal acts which symbolically hurt the other or the use of threats to hurt the other" (Straus, 1979, p. 79). Compare this tactic with that of reasoning which involves discussing issues calmly, obtaining additional information about the conflict, or seeking outside help for a problem. In addition, physical aggression and violence as conflict resolution tactics include severe abuse involving pushing, slapping, hitting, or threatening a partner with a knife or gun, which all potentially may result in a great deal of physical harm.

Lesbians who use physical aggression and violence as a means of conflict resolution tend to overly depend on their partners and, hence, resort to violence to inhibit their partners' effort to be independent (Renzetti, 1988). Dependency also has been linked to self-destructive behaviors such as alcohol abuse in lesbian communities (Nicoloff & Stigletz, 1987).

Battering among lesbians has been defined as a "pattern of violent or coercive behavior whereby a lesbian seeks to control the thoughts, beliefs or conduct of her intimate partner or to punish the intimate for resisting the perpetrator's control" (Hart, 1986, p. 173). Battering threats may be direct, but often these threats are indirect or veiled efforts at intimidation used to establish control and power over the battered partner. Consequently, when the battered lesbian responds with increased fear, efforts to change the batterer's behavior, or attempts to distance herself from the relationship, the batterer's control, power, and battering escalate (Hammond, 1989). This pattern of control, intimidation and escalation of violence also characterizes violent and abusive heterosexual relationships (Straus, Gelles, & Steinmetz, 1980).

Hypothesis 2 in this study was that *lesbians who report higher levels of fusion will use more verbal and physical aggression and violence strategies but fewer reasoning strategies for conflict resolution.* Hart (1986) indicated that lesbians who use physical aggression and violence as a means of conflict resolution do so to dominate and to achieve compliance from their partner. They express feelings of powerlessness and helplessness in their relationships, viewing independent and self-caring actions by their partner as sources of conflict and a means of being controlled by their partner. Lesbian batterers see themselves as victims. Consequently, they use violence to gain control over themselves and their partners (Hart, 1986; Renzetti, 1988).

Fusion and Self-Esteem

In merged couples, couple harmony may become the primary issue so that partners deny differences and avoid, rather than resolve, conflict. Individual differences, interests, activities, and friendships are relinquished (Krestan & Bepko, 1980; Pearlman, 1989). Prolonged fusion demands individual compromise and loss of self. This loss frequently is accompanied by anger, feelings of powerlessness and low self-esteem (Pearlman, 1989). Hence, in the current study, Hypothesis 3 was that *lesbians with higher levels of fusion in their relationships will report lower levels of self-esteem and independence as personality traits.*

METHODOLOGY

Sample

The lesbian participants in the current study were women who attended a large regional women's music festival held in the Southeast. Of 400 questionnaires distributed, 275 were returned, for a response rate of 69%. Respondents were guaranteed confidentiality. Each respondent was, or had been during the previous 6 months, involved in a lesbian relationship.

Instruments

The following variables were measured: fusion, conflict resolution tactics, sources of conflict, personality traits, and self-esteem.

Fusion. Fusion was measured by six items. On a 5-point Likert-type scale of 1 (never) to 5 (always), with higher scores indicating more fusion, each respondent was asked how often she felt the need to share recreational and social activities, felt the need to do everything together, felt the need for independent time with friends, insisted on sharing professional services, made regular phone calls at work, and insisted on sharing monies and clothing.

A factor analysis of the fusion items produced two subscales. Items relating to sharing recreational and social time, feeling the need to share everything, and needing independent time with friends form a subscale labeled *fusion time issues.* The reliability (Cronbach's alpha) of this subscale was .89. The second subscale, labeled *sharing,* contains items that focused on sharing concrete items and services (e.g., monies, clothes, professional services, and phone calls). The reliability of this subscale was .79.

Conflict resolution tactics. Straus's (1979) Conflict Resolution Tactics Scale was used to measure the nature and extent of reasoning, verbal aggression, physical aggression, and physical violence used to resolve conflicts. The Conflict Resolution Tactics Scale has 19 items, and respondents used a Likert scale of 0 (never) to 6 (more than 20 times a year) to respond to how often each item was used as a means of conflict resolution. The subscale labeled *reasoning* includes resolution strategies such as discussing, getting information, and asking for help outside the relationship. Reliability for this subscale was .54.

Verbal aggression includes verbal and nonverbal acts in which one person symbolically hurts the other. Acts include making threats, sulking and refusing to talk, stomping out, and saying something to spite the partner. The reliability for the verbal aggression subscale was high: .84. The items composing the physical aggression subscale have been described as mild forms of physical abuse (e.g., throwing an object at a partner, pushing, shoving, or slapping). Reliability was .90. The violence subscale carries high risk for the victim and includes kicking, hitting, beating, as well as threatening to use knife or gun. The reliability for the violence subscale was .96.

Sources of conflict. Almost an infinite number of issues can serve as possible sources of conflict for persons in intimate relationships. Based on typical sources of conflict identified in the conflict and family violence literature (Hart, 1986; Straus, 1979), the authors of the current study developed a list of 26 potential sources of conflict. Respondents used a Likert scale of 0 (never) to 3 (nearly all the time) to respond to how often they had conflicts over the listed items.

Three subscales were formed from these 26 sources. A subscale of *external conflicts* includes issues related to employment status, jobs, and how money is spent. Reliability for this subscale was .66. The *internal conflicts* subscale includes emotional and financial dependency of both the respondent and her partner, jealousy, and drug and alcohol use. Reliability for this subscale was .73. The third subscale comprises tasks performed in relationships as well as other *relational issues* such as housekeeping, cooking, children, relatives, friends, and sexual activities. Reliability for this subscale was .80.

Personality traits. Lesbians in the sample were asked to describe themselves and their partner by using a list of six personality traits reflecting autonomy. Traits were placed at opposite ends of a continuum (i.e., "not at all dependent" to "very dependent"). A Likert type scale of 1 (strongly disagree) to 5 (strongly agree) was used to form the extremes of the continuum. The scale consists of traits such as like feeling not at all independent, feeling submissive, being passive, needing other people's approval, having one's feelings hurt easily, not feeling confident, and giving up easily. The reliability of this subscale was .67.

Self-Esteem. Hudson's (1982) Index of Self-Esteem was designed to measure the degree or severity of the problem the respondent has with self-esteem. A high score on the Index of Self-Esteem indicates the respondent has a problem with self-esteem. The 25-item scale includes items such as "I feel that people would not like me if they really knew me well," "I feel that I bore people," and "I feel I get pushed around more than others." This index has an alpha coefficient of .93.

Analysis

Data were analyzed using 95% confidence intervals (CI) and Pearson product-moment correlations. The level of significance was set at $p < .05$. Composite variables were subjected to exploratory factor analyses (varimax rotation). Reliabilities (Cronbach's alpha) were computed for all composite scales.

RESULTS

Research Question

The research question addressed the extent of fusion within the sample. The fusion scale used in the study contained the subscales *fusion time issues* and *sharing*. Participants reported overall moderate levels of fusion. Confidence intervals were used to determine an expected range for means. If confidence levels do not overlap, they may be considered significantly different. Respondents ($N = 275$)

reported more time fusion (X = 2.80, $p < .05$, $SD = .89$, $t(271) = 8.69$, $p = > .001$), than sharing fusion (X = 2.28, $p < .05$, $SD = .79$). (These two variables could range from 1.00 to 5.00). Time fusion and sharing fusion also were directly correlated, $r = .33$, $p < .01$, such that participants who reported high time fusion tended to report high sharing fusion.

Tests of Hypotheses

Hypothesis 1. The first hypothesis proposed that higher levels of fusion will relate to more internal and relational conflicts and less external conflicts; this hypothesis was partially supported. Correlations among the three groupings of conflict sources (internal, external, and relational) were run with the fusion scales. Time fusion was not significantly related to reports of internal ($r = .03$) or relational ($r = .08$) sources of conflict. Time fusion, however, was directly correlated with external sources of conflict ($r = .12$, $p < .01$). That is, participants who reported time fusion were likely to report more external sources of conflict.

The relations for sharing fusion were slightly different. Sharing fusion was directly related to reported internal ($r = .17$, $p < .01$), relational ($r = .13$, $p < .01$), and external ($r = .20$, $p < .01$) sources of conflict. That is, participants who reported high sharing fusion tended to report more of all sources of conflict.

Hypothesis 2. The second hypothesis proposed that with increased levels of fusion, there would be more verbal and physical aggression, as well as violence used as conflict strategies, with less use of reasoning strategies. This hypothesis, which was partially supported, was tested using a series of correlations among the two fusion scales (fusion time issues and sharing) and the four conflict resolution strategies (reasoning, verbal aggression, physical aggression, and violence).

For the time dimension of the fusion scale, time fusion was related only to verbal and physical aggression as conflict resolutions. Participants who reported high time fusion reported using more verbal aggression strategies ($r = .14$, $p < .01$) and more physical aggression strategies ($r = .11$, $p < .05$). Time fusion was not significantly related to reasoning strategies of conflict resolution ($r = -.05$) or to violence ($r = .03$).

The sharing dimension of fusion was significantly correlated with all four conflict resolution strategies. That is, participants who reported high sharing fusion tended to report more frequent use of reasoning ($r = .10$, $p < .05$), verbal aggression ($r = .18$, $p < .01$), physical aggression ($r = .19$, $p < .01$), and violence ($r = .17$, $p < .01$) as styles of conflict resolution. This finding may reflect more overall conflict or simply more aggressive forms of conflict resolution because the reasoning correlation was the weakest.

Related to self-esteem and violence, a finding that was not predicted indicated that lesbians with low self-esteem reported using higher levels of verbal and physical aggression as well as violence to resolve conflicts. This is consistent with literature that reports profiles of batterers and victims in heterosexual relationships (Gelles & Cornell, 1985).

Hypothesis 3. The third hypothesis predicted that reports of higher fusion will relate to lower self-esteem and lower levels of independence as a personality trait. This hypothesis was partially supported. Self-esteem was inversely related to scores on sharing fusion ($r = -.10$, $p < .01$). That is, participants who reported high sharing fusion tended to have lower self-esteem. Self-esteem and time fusion, however, were not significantly related ($r = .03$). That is, scores on time fusion were unrelated to self-esteem.

Independence was not significantly related to either time fusion ($r = -.04$) or sharing fusion ($r = -.05$). That is, participants' ratings of independence were unrelated to scores on fusion. Independence was also related to other variables in ways not predicted. Independence was directly correlated with self-esteem ($r = .40$, $p < .001$) such that high scores on independence were related to high self-esteem. Independence was also directly correlated with both physical ($r = .14$, $p < .01$) and violent ($r = .23$, $p < .01$) conflict strategies but inversely correlated with crisis strategies ($r = .08$, $p < .01$).

DISCUSSION

Several of the proposed hypotheses in the investigation were confirmed. Many of the correlations were statistically significant due to the large sample size; however, most were small in magnitude. The extent of fusion in lesbian relationships from a nonclinical population was not reported as being excessive. Rather, moderate levels of fusion were reported. This finding differs from a number of previous works that documented high levels of fusion (Berg-Cross, 1988; Krestan & Bepko, 1980; Pearlman, 1989). Although all close relationships require a balancing of the desire for intimacy and the desire for autonomy (Peplau, Cochran, Rook, & Padesky, 1978), emotional attachment has been found to be highly valued in lesbian relationships (Schneider, 1986).

Only one article was found that questioned whether enmeshment was a value-laden term. Zacks, Green, and Marrow (1988) expressed concern that the concept of enmeshment evolved from traditional male-oriented biases that value independence and clear boundaries in relationships. These characteristics may be norms for heterosexual couples, but perhaps the qualities desired in lesbian relationships vary from those desired in heterosexual relationships. One such difference may be the level of fusion that is functional in women-oriented relationships. Consequently, social workers may need to look closely at their own comfort level with a couple's closeness. McCandlish (1985) suggested that traditional heterosexual therapists may feel uncomfortable with the level of closeness in a lesbian relationship, and thus may view that relationship as immature and pathological, contributing to the couple's separation.

Furthermore, high time fusion appeared to be less problematic than high sharing fusion. One possible explanation may be that lesbians simply enjoy spending large amounts of time with their partners and participating in social activities together. Lesbian couples may reconcile issues of sharing time and space more easily than heterosexual couples. Apparently, this allocation of time does not cause conflict in the lesbian relationship nor contribute to the loss of oneself. This finding is consistent with the Peplau, Cochran, Rook, and Padesky (1978) finding that lesbians reported being in close, loving relationships and also reported high levels of satisfaction. Perhaps one of the strengths of a lesbian relationship lies in the value both partners place on relating. Women who have previously related to men have often reported a sense of relief that the burden of keeping the relationship intimate, close, and vital was no longer solely their responsibility. Their lesbian partner often accepts equal responsibility for the closeness of the relationship.

High levels of sharing fusion, however, do appear to affect one's sense of personal autonomy. Respondents who reported high sharing fusion also reported lower self-esteem, more conflict in the relationship, and poorer conflict resolution strategies. Lesbians who reported low self-esteem also reported higher levels of fusion relating to the sharing of concrete items (money and clothes) and the sharing of professional services. One possible explanation for this finding is that people's choice of possessions (e.g., clothing and automobiles) is in many ways a statement about personal identity. Those possessions indicate to the larger world how people view themselves and project their individuality. Sharing of these items and maintaining appropriate boundaries is more difficult than sharing large amounts of time together.

Participants who reported high–not moderate–time fusion also reported high sharing fusion. Although both types of fusion were related to verbal and physical aggression as a means of conflict resolution, respondents who reported high sharing fusion also reported more frequent use of violence to resolve conflicts. But both time fusion and sharing fusion were positively correlated with verbal and physical aggression. Also, sharing fusion was positively correlated with violence. M. Wilder (personal communication, October 13, 1993), in her work with lesbian domestic violence perpetrators, indicated problematic issues involving negotiating boundaries for both sharing of time and possessions (e.g., clothes, money, or car). Clients who have difficulty expressing their needs eventually become so frustrated they use physical aggression to resolve conflict. She further stated that when a client has high levels of both time and sharing fusion, the prognosis for change is more difficult.

Future research should more fully identify the strengths as well as the problematic aspects of high levels of closeness in intimate lesbian relationships, both sexual and platonic. For example, what are the boundary issues with two women who are not sexually involved? Future studies of lesbian relationships should further explore issues of fusion and conflict resolution.

REFERENCES

Berg-Cross, L. (1988). Lesbians, family process and individuation. *Journal of College Student Psychotherapy, 3*(1), 97-112.

Burch, B. (1982). Psychological merger in lesbian couples: A joint ego psychological and systems approach. *Family Therapy, 9*(3), 201-208.

Caldwell, M., & Peplau, L. A. (1984). The balance of power in lesbian relationships. *Sex Roles, 10*(7/8), 587-599.

Canary, D. J., Cunningham, E. M., & Cody, M. J. (1988). Goal types, gender, and locus of control in managing interpersonal conflict. *Communication Research, 15*(4), 426-446.

Chodorow, N. (1978). *The reproduction of mothering: Psychoanalysis and the sociology of gender.* Berkeley: University of California Press.

Covey, S. (1989). *The seven habits of highly effective people.* New York: Simon and Schuster.

Douglas, C. (1990). *Counseling same-sex couples.* New York: Norton Press.

Eldridge, N., & Gilbert, L. (1990). Correlates of relationship satisfaction in lesbian couples. *Psychology of Women Quarterly, 14*, 43-62.

Gelles, R., & Cornell, C. (1985). *Intimate violence in families.* Beverly Hills, CA: Sage.

Gelles, R., & Straus, M. (1978). Determinants of violence in the family: Toward a theoretical integration. In R. Gelles & M. Strauss (Eds.), *Contemporary theories about the family* (pp. 549-581). New York: Free Press.

Hammond, N. (1989). Lesbian victims of relationship violence. *Journal of Interpersonal Violence, 4*, 89-105.

Hart, B. (1986). Lesbian battering: An examination. In K. Lobel (Ed.), *Naming the violence: Speaking out about lesbian violence* (pp. 173-189). Seattle, WA: Seal Press.

Hocker, J. L., & Wilmot, W. W. (1985). *Interpersonal conflict.* Dubuque, IA: William C. Brown.

Hudson, W. (1982). *The clinical measurement package: A field manual.* Chicago: Dorsey Press.

Krestan, J., & Bepko, C. (1980). The problem of fusion in the lesbian relationship. *Family Process, 19*, 277-289.

Kurdek, L. (1992). Relationship stability and relationship satisfaction in cohabiting gay and lesbian couples: A prospective longitudinal test of the contextual and interdependence models. *Journal of Social and Personal Relationships, 9*, 125-142.

Lerner, H. G. (1989). *The dance of intimacy.* New York: Harper & Row.

Lindenbaum, J. (1980). The shattering of an illusion: The problem of competition in lesbian relationships. *Feminist Studies, 11*(1), 85-103.

Lloyd, S. A. (1990). A behavioral self-report technique for assessing conflict in close relationships. *Journal of Social and Personal Relationships, 7*, 265-272.

McCandlish, D. (1985). Therapeutic issues with lesbian couples. *Journal of Homosexuality, 7*(1), 71-78.

Minuchin, S. (1974). *Families and family therapy.* Cambridge: Harvard University Press.

Nicoloff, L., & Stigletz, E. (1987). Lesbian alcoholism: Etiology, treatment, and recovery. In the Boston Lesbian Psychologies Collectives (Ed.), *Lesbian psychologies* (pp. 283-293). Urbana: University of Illinois Press.

Pearlman, S. (1989). Distancing and connectedness: Impact on couples formation in lesbian relationships. *Women & Therapy, 9*(3), 77-88.

Peplau, L. A., Cochran, S., Rook, K., & Padesky, C. (1978). Loving women: Attachment and autonomy in lesbian relationships. *Journal of Social Issues, 34*(3), 7-27.

Peplau, L.A., Padesky, C., & Hamilton, M. (1983). Satisfaction in lesbian relationships. *Journal of Homosexuality, 8*(2), 23-35.

Renzetti, C. (1988). Violence in lesbian relationships: A preliminary analysis of causal factors. *Journal of Interpersonal Violence, 3*(4), 381-399.

Roloff, M. (1987). Communication and conflict. In C. R. Berger & S. H. Chaffee (Eds.), *Handbook of communication science* (pp. 69-76). Newbury Park, CA: Sage.

Schneider, N. (1986). The relationships of cohabiting lesbian and heterosexual couples: A comparison. *Psychology of Women Quarterly, 10*, 234-239.

Sillars, A. L. (1980). Attributions and communications in roommate conflicts. *Communication Monographs, 47*, 180-200.

Straus, M. (1979). Measuring intrafamily conflict and violence: The conflict tactics (CT) scale. *Journal of Marriage and the Family, 41*, 75-88.

Straus, M., Gelles, R., & Steinmetz, S. (1980). *Behind closed doors: Violence in American families.* Garden City, NY: Doubleday.

Zacks, E., Green, R. J., & Marrow, J. (1988). Comparing lesbian and heterosexual couples on the circumplex model: An initial investigation. *Family Process, 27*, 471-484.

Index

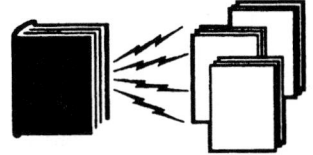

Haworth
DOCUMENT DELIVERY
SERVICE

This new service provides a single-article order form for any article from a Haworth journal.

- *Time Saving:* No running around from library to library to find a specific article.
- *Cost Effective:* All costs are kept down to a minimum.
- *Fast Delivery:* Choose from several options, including same-day FAX.
- *No Copyright Hassles:* You will be supplied by the original publisher.
- *Easy Payment:* Choose from several easy payment methods.

Open Accounts Welcome for ...
- Library Interlibrary Loan Departments
- Library Network/Consortia Wishing to Provide Single-Article Services
- Indexing/Abstracting Services with Single Article Provision Services
- Document Provision Brokers and Freelance Information Service Providers

---

MAIL or *FAX* THIS ENTIRE ORDER FORM TO:

Haworth Document Delivery Service
The Haworth Press, Inc.
10 Alice Street
Binghamton, NY 13904-1580

or FAX: (607) 722-6362
or CALL: 1-800-3-HAWORTH
(1-800-342-9678; 9am-5pm EST)

PLEASE SEND ME PHOTOCOPIES OF THE FOLLOWING SINGLE ARTICLES:

1) Journal Title: _____

   Vol/Issue/Year: _____ Starting & Ending Pages: _____

   Article Title: _____

   _____

2) Journal Title: _____

   Vol/Issue/Year: _____ Starting & Ending Pages: _____

   Article Title: _____

   _____

3) Journal Title: _____

   Vol/Issue/Year: _____ Starting & Ending Pages: _____

   Article Title: _____

   _____

4) Journal Title: _____

   Vol/Issue/Year: _____ Starting & Ending Pages: _____

   Article Title: _____

(See other side for Costs and Payment Information)

COSTS: Please figure your cost to order quality copies of an article.

1. Set-up charge per article: $8.00

        ($8.00 × number of separate articles)   _____

2. Photocopying charge for each article:

        1-10 pages: $1.00   _____

        11-19 pages: $3.00   _____

        20-29 pages: $5.00   _____

        30+ pages: $2.00/10 pages   _____

3. Flexicover (optional): $2.00/article   _____

4. Postage & Handling: US: $1.00 for the first article/

        $.50 each additional article   _____

        Federal Express: $25.00   _____

        Outside US: $2.00 for first article/

        $.50 each additional article _____

5. Same-day FAX service: $.35 per page   _____

        GRAND TOTAL: _____

METHOD OF PAYMENT: (please check one)

❑ Check enclosed   ❑ Please ship and bill. PO # _____

        (sorry we can ship and bill to bookstores only! All others must pre-pay)

❑ Charge to my credit card: ❑ Visa; ❑ MasterCard; ❑ American Express;

Account Number:_____ Expiration date:_____

Signature: ✗_____

Name: _____ Institution: _____

Address: _____

_____

City: _____ State:_____ Zip:_____

Phone Number: _____ FAX Number: _____

MAIL or *FAX* THIS ENTIRE ORDER FORM TO:

Haworth Document Delivery Service	**or FAX:** (607) 722-6362
The Haworth Press, Inc.	**or CALL:** 1-800-3-HAWORTH
10 Alice Street	(1-800-342-9678; 9am-5pm EST)
Binghamton, NY 13904-1580	